THE COMPLETE BOOK OF TRADITIONAL REIKI

"Amy Rowland's book is an engaging story of discovery, which has been a pleasure to read. Contains well-researched knowledge of Reiki's origins and reveals practical and metaphysical insights into its use and effectiveness today."

CHRIS PARKES AND PENNY PARKES, REIKI MASTERS
AND COAUTHORS OF *15-MINUTE REIKI*

Praise for Amy Rowland's previous book, *Reiki for the Heart and Soul*

"*Reiki for the Heart and Soul* is a gift to us from a remarkable woman who lives and breathes her work. The book literally loves us into each and every precious principle, weaving it's magic as we read, bringing us into a deeper understanding. I feel it should be required reading for all dedicated practitioners and teachers."

MARI HALL, FOUNDER AND DIRECTOR OF INTERNATIONAL ASSOCIATION
FOR REIKI AND AUTHOR OF *REIKI FOR THE SOUL: THE ELEVENTH DOOR*

"This is a well-written Reiki book that weaves together many important details with a wonderful spiritual sentiment. It grounds one in the here and now and inspires practitioners to look deeply into their own healing and to help others."

WILLIAM LEE RAND, AUTHOR OF *REIKI: THE HEALING TOUCH* AND DIRECTOR OF THE
INTERNATIONAL CENTER FOR REIKI TRAINING

THE
COMPLETE
BOOK
OF TRADITIONAL
REIKI

PRACTICAL METHODS
FOR PERSONAL
AND PLANETARY
HEALING

AMY Z. ROWLAND

Healing Arts Press

Rochester, Vermont • Toronto, Canada

Healing Arts Press
One Park Street
Rochester, Vermont 05767
www.HealingArtsPress.com

Healing Arts Press is a division of Inner Traditions International

Note to the reader: This book is intended as an informational guide. The remedies, approaches, and techniques described herein are meant to supplement, and not to be a substitute for, professional medical care or treatment. They should not be used to treat a serious ailment without prior consultation with a qualified health care professional.

LIBRARY OF CONGRESS CATALOGING-IN-PUBLICATION DATA

Rowland, Amy Zaffarano.
  The complete book of traditional reiki : practical methods for personal and planetary healing / Amy Z. Rowland.
      p. cm.
  Summary: "A comprehensive guide to the hands-on healing techniques taught to practitioners in a traditional Reiki I class"—Provided by publisher.
  Rev ed. of: Traditional reiki for our times. c1998.
  Includes bibliographical references and index.
  ISBN 978-1-59477-351-8 (pbk.)
  1. Reiki (Healing system) I. Rowland, Amy Zaffarano. Traditional reiki for our times. II. Title.
  RZ403.R45R68 2010
  615.8'51—dc22
                                                                    2010004912

Printed and bound in the United States by the P. A. Hutchison Company

10 9 8 7 6 5 4 3 2 1

Text design and layout by Priscilla Baker
This book was typeset in Berkeley with Amadeus used as a display typeface

Photographs of Mikao Usui's gravesite by Elyssa Matthews
Photographs of Usui Memorial by Elyssa Matthews and Daniela Tudor
Translation of the text of the Usui Memorial into English by Rev. Hyakuten Inamoto
Computer-generated image of the Gainen provided by Dave King
Photographs of Amy Levin, Yvonne DeVastey, and Donna Fasano by Donna Glas
Photographs of Mikao Usui, Chujiro Hayashi, and Hawayo Takata are considered to be in the public domain; print images supplied by William Rand. The image of Mrs. Hawayo Takata's master certificate, filed in the offices of the City and County of Honolulu, is in the public domain.
Illustrations by Rita Zaffarano

For the highest good of all concerned

CONTENTS

REIKI LEVEL I

REIKI LEVEL II AND BEYOND

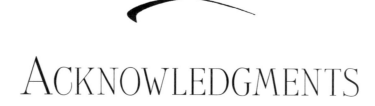

ACKNOWLEDGMENTS

The opportunity to review and to revise a book so that it remains meaning-ful to readers is rare and precious. I am grateful to Jon Graham at Healing Arts Press, an imprint of Inner Traditions • Bear & Company, for saying "yes" to my e-mailed query, and to everyone on staff who worked to put this new edition of *Traditional Reiki for Our Times* into your hands.

Since my primary purpose in revising the book has been to update the his-tory presented, I want to thank all those who have been involved in research on Reiki's origins in Japan, Hawaii, and elsewhere, in particular Frank Arjava Petter and William Rand; I commend those who sponsored Mr. Hiroshi Doi and Reverend Hyakuten Inamoto on their first and subsequent trips from Japan to the West to share information about Reiki techniques practiced within the Usui Reiki Ryoho Gakkai, the learning society established by Mikao Usui in the 1920s; and I feel a debt of gratitude to Mr. Kondor, Chairperson of the Gakkai, who has kindly given permission for this cultural exchange.

I regard Mr. Doi and Rev. Inamoto as among my most important spiritual teachers. I appreciate Mr. Doi's groundbreaking book, *Iyashino Gendai Reiki-ho (Modern Reiki Method for Healing)* as an effort to present Reiki in a way that will bridge cultures; I am thankful to the American, British, and Canadian Reiki masters who ensured the book's translation into English, and all of those involved in the translation process. I am grateful to Tom Rigler for teaching me the historical Usui Reiki Ryoho techniques and modern Gendai Reiki, as he learned both from Mr. Doi, and to Rev. Inamoto for teaching me Komyo Reiki, his synthesis of the Western and Japanese styles of Reiki.

The Complete Book of Traditional Reiki features some new photos and images to support the explanation of Reiki history. The beautiful photos of the Usui gravesite and memorial by Canadian Reiki Master Elyssa Matthews and one of her students, Daniela Tudor, make me want to join them on their next trip to Japan, at cherry blossom time. Rev. Inamoto has kindly granted permission for use of his translation of the inscription on the Usui Memorial into English, making the story of the life of Mikao Usui, as remembered and recorded by his students a year after his death, accessible to us today. Dave King has provided a computer-generated image of the Gainen, the original Reiki principles, from double titles to closing, allowing readers to get a sense of the orderly progression of the precepts as pathwork. My deepest thanks to all of you!

David Gleekel and John Graybill, thank you for all of your support and friendship through the years, and for connecting me to potential translators. Dave King, thank you for the gift of your friendship. Your dedication, patience, and wisdom awe me. Mark Clutton, thank you for checking in on me so often via transatlantic phone calls. You have encouraged me in my writing and in my spiritual pathwork. Ellen Phillips, thank you for talking writing and Reiki with me over so many cups of coffee through the years. You have reminded me to pace myself and stay in balance.

Reiki remains the greatest blessing of my life. I will always be grateful to Angela Rapalyea and Bruce and Estelle Rausch, who introduced me to this experience and helped me to connect to my first teacher, Rev. Beth Gray. The gratitude I feel to Beth and to Frank DuGan, and through their instruction and inspiration, to Hawayo Takata, Chujiro Hayashi, and Mikao Usui, is beyond expression in words: I honor them for their courage, dedication, and commitment, and I thank them for their endless patience and compassion for this student, still learning so many lessons each day.

My sense of Reiki would not be so complete or clear without the joyful sharing of stories by fellow students and practitioners, and by my own students and clients, who will hear the echoes of their voices and laughter in the pages of this book. Their stories, and those of my fellow Reiki masters, continue to be a catalyst for the evolution of my understanding and the deepening of my love for this energy, which is the true teacher and healer of us all.

The support of family and friends has been essential to the creation and completion of this book, and a source of comfort to me as well. I particularly want to thank Amy Levin, Yvonne DeVastey, and Donna Fasano, the models for the photographs demonstrating hand positions; Donna Glas, the photographer; and Rita Zaffarano, the artist (and my mother!), for contributing their loving energy, their patience, and their smiles to this undertaking. Donna Fasano and Janet Kuchler reviewed sections of the manuscript, as did Nicholas Chin and Ton't Lam, offering insightful suggestions for improvement and encouragement to me on those days when I felt overwhelmed. Online friends, too many to name, sent me distant healing as I needed it, offered essential words of support, and reminded me, again and again, to be guided only by God within me.

I also wish to thank the global community of Reiki practitioners and Reiki masters who meet and talk with one another via the Internet. I commend the spirit of open inquiry, of service, and of tolerance for differences evident in so many blogs, posts to forums, and across so many websites. I am grateful for your honesty, your integrity, your commitment to healing. Thank you for freely sharing information, inspired words, and emerging vision.

Special thanks to all those who assisted me in my research on nontraditional and emerging forms of Reiki for the first edition of this book: Marsha Burack, Tsy Ford, Earlene Gleisner, Robert Henley, Gary Lightfield, Douglas Morris, Suzanne Parnell, William Rand, Sharon Wendt, and Patrick Zeigler. I appreciate your courtesy, your clarity, your patience, and your encouragement. I value your efforts to educate the world community about Reiki.

I also want to thank Jamaica Burns, my editor for *The Complete Book of Traditional Reiki,* and Susan Davidson, my original editor at Healing Arts Press. Both of you have worked with me and with the manuscript in a caring and thoughtful way. I appreciate your patience, sensitivity and insight, and strong editorial skills. I remain confident that everyone at Healing Arts Press will shepherd this revised edition of *Traditional Reiki for Our Times* into the hands of those readers who will most benefit from reading it.

Finally, my thanks to those who read this book with an open mind and heart and a willingness to consider the possibility that healing may occur more quickly, more deeply, and with more lasting effect than we often expect; and sometimes, where there is little or no hope. May your reward be to witness miracles.

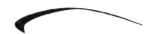

PREFACE TO THE REVISED EDITION

Authors are not often granted the opportunity to update and to revise a book, but this particular book, since it was first published in 1998 as *Traditional Reiki for Our Times,* has proven to be of help to those considering learning Reiki; to newly trained practitioners who want to recall and to reflect on the lessons of their Reiki I class; and to those teaching a basic course in Usui Shiki Ryoho. It has been made available not only in English, but also in Lithuanian, Spanish, Portuguese, and Russian, and has sparked conversations about Reiki across continents. To everyone who has found the first edition of this book of value, I express my deepest thanks. I hope that the revised edition, which you now hold in your hands, will offer you a helpful, new perspective on traditional Reiki that enables you to see how it has evolved into one of the most important complementary medicine practices in the world today.

Now, as before, I take very seriously my responsibility to describe clearly, in book form, the very thorough training provided by my teacher, Hawayo Takata–trained Reiki Master Rev. Beth Gray (April 11, 1918–May 13, 2008), in the basic course in Usui Shiki Reiki Ryoho. This traditional form of Reiki (sometimes called "Western Reiki") was first taught outside Japan in 1937, in the Territory of Hawaii, by Dr. Chujiro Hayashi, with the assistance of his master level student, Mrs. Hawayo Takata. He certified her to teach in February 1938, and she opened her first healing center in Kauai almost

immediately. Through her work in Hawaii, treating clients, she "cured"*
many people, evolved simpler treatment methods, and developed an unwavering trust in the energy she had come to know so well. In the 1970s, during the last decade of her life, Takata decided to focus more on teaching all levels of Reiki; she also trained twenty-two Reiki masters to ensure that the Usui system of Reiki healing would not be lost. As a result of this very wise decision, Usui Shiki Reiki Ryoho (also referred to throughout this book as "traditional Reiki" or Western Reiki) has become the most widely practiced and taught form in the world—countless millions of practitioners, from America and Australia to New Zealand and Zimbabwe, are now empowered to offer Reiki healing. To share my understanding of this traditional form of Reiki with you is a privilege. To share some of my memories of my teacher, Rev. Beth Gray, with you is a joy.

Yet there are good reasons to revise some chapters of the first edition. In the dozen years that have elapsed since the book's publication, much new information about Reiki's origins has come to light. Researchers in Japan have located and visited Taniai Mura (now named Miyamacho[1]), the town in which Mikao Usui, the founder of Reiki, was born in August 1865, as well as the cemetery outside Saihoji Temple in Tokyo where some of his ashes are interred. They have searched for the location of the original Usui Reiki Ryoho Gakkai, the learning society he founded in Tokyo, as well as the clinic established by Dr. Chujiro Hayashi, Usui's student, in the Shinano-machi section[2] of the same city, at Usui's direction. (This is the Reiki clinic where Hawayo Takata was treated for her various ailments in 1935 and where, after her recovery, she trained as a Reiki practitioner under Hayashi's supervision, between 1935 and 1937.) And many Reiki practitioners and teachers from around the world, like pilgrims, have now retraced Mikao Usui's footsteps to the top of Mount Kurama, to see where he sat in meditation, hoping to experience enlightenment, and have visited Saihoji Temple, to place offerings at his grave.

Researchers in Japan have also discovered texts and documents that enable the story of Reiki to be told more fully. Beside Usui's grave is the Usui Memorial,

---

*Hawayo Takata herself uses the word "cured" in one of her early unpublished diary entries (May 1, 1937); most traditional Reiki masters make a point of telling new practitioners that it is universal life-force energy, channeled through the practitioner's hands that cures, not the practitioner himself.

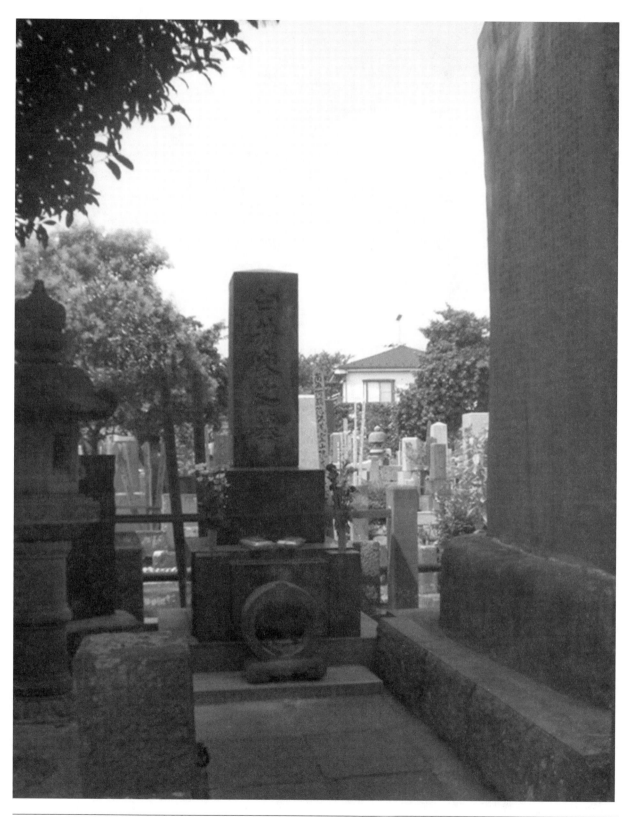

Mikao Usui's ashes are interred in a cemetery outside Saihoji Temple in Tokyo. Reiki practitioners and teachers from around the world visit his grave to burn incense, leave offerings, and say prayers of gratitude.

a tall stone inscribed with a long text hailing him as a great spiritual teacher and healer and describing a few of the important events of his life. Included within this text is the Gainen, a more complete version of the five familiar statements Mrs. Takata and the Reiki masters that she trained introduced to the world as the Reiki principles ("Just for today, do not worry. / Just for today, do not anger. / Be grateful. Count your blessings. / Do an honest day's work. / Be kind to all living things."*) Bracketed by a double title, "The Secret Method of Inviting Happiness / The Miraculous Medicine for All Diseases," and Mikao Usui's recommendation to focus on the principles in meditation, these guidelines for daily life now take on new significance.

Other important primary and secondary source materials have surfaced through the efforts of researchers and the generosity of today's Usui Reiki Ryoho Gakkai. The text of the Hikkei, the manual used by Mikao Usui to teach beginners, has been translated multiple times and become a subject of ongoing study. (The book contains a table of contents; the Gainen or Reiki principles; Usui's explanation of Reiki presented in question and answer form; a list of recommended hand positions for the treatment of particular illnesses and medical conditions; and selected *waka,* inspirational poems composed by the Meiji Emperor.) A few new photographs of Mikao Usui, alone and with some of his followers gathered around him, have been published in books and made available online.

The comparable manual used by Dr. Chujiro Hayashi has also been translated into English numerous times and made available for study. Tadao Yamaguchi, who learned Reiki from his mother, Chiyoko Yamaguchi (1921–2003), one of Dr. Hayashi's students, presents additional information about Dr. Hayashi and his teaching methods, and several previously unpublished photographs, in *Light on the Origins of Reiki: A Handbook for Practicing the Original Reiki of Usui and Hayashi.* Tadao Yamaguchi now teaches Jikiden Reiki with the intention of "pass[ing] on the original teachings of Hayashi Sensei."[3] His book makes it possible to compare Hayashi's teaching methods and the techniques

---

*This version of the Reiki principles is the one that I was taught by my teacher, Rev. Beth Gray; other versions, very similar in wording, were presented by Takata to other students. For more about these variations and about the Reiki principles, please see *Reiki for the Heart and Soul: The Reiki Principles as Spiritual Pathwork* (Rochester, Vt.: Inner Traditions, 2008).

he demonstrated with those of Mikao Usui; in addition, it invites the reader to reconsider Takata's teaching methods as an evolution of Hayashi's, adapted for a Western audience.

How do we know how Mikao Usui taught? Since 1999, Japanese Reiki Master Hiroshi Doi has traveled worldwide, with the permission of the present-day Usui Reiki Ryoho Gakkai, presenting the history of Reiki, as it is understood in his homeland, and demonstrating Usui Reiki Ryoho (traditional Japanese) techniques, at international conferences, workshops, and classes. Mr. Doi also provides instruction in Gendai Reiki, a modern synthesis of traditional Japanese and Western Reiki. Zen Buddhist priest Hyakuten Inamoto, who has often accompanied Mr. Doi on his travels, offers another fresh perspective. Rev. Inamoto, after studying with Mrs. Yamaguchi for a year, as well as Mr. Doi, now teaches Komyo Reiki, another modern synthesis of traditional techniques that emphasizes Reiki's spiritual nature.

Research in Hawaii, home of Hawayo Takata, the first Western Reiki master, has produced photos of her former home and clinic in Hilo.[4] In addition, her Reiki Master Certificate, signed and dated February 21, 1938, by Dr. Chujiro Hayashi, witnessed by Yoshio Hanao, and filed in the offices of the City of Honolulu, has now been published in books and online. Dr. Hayashi clearly intended that Takata's qualifications to teach Reiki be made a matter of public record. The story of his trip to Hawaii with his daughter and their six-month stay to help Takata establish Reiki in the Territory of Hawaii is told by her authorized biographer, Helen J. Haberly, in *Reiki: Hawayo Takata's Story*[5] and by Takata-trained Reiki Master Fran Brown, in *Living Reiki: Takata's Teachings.*[6]

This wealth of resources, new and old, is very helpful in "setting the record straight" on some of the details of Mikao Usui's life and the early history of Reiki as a healing and spiritual practice in Japan. Some of these details contradict the story of Reiki published in the first edition of this book, which was a retelling of the story told by my teacher, Rev. Beth Gray, who first heard it from Takata in 1974.[7] Japanese Reiki masters say that, contrary to Takata's story, Mikao Usui did *not* teach at a Christian school for boys; he did *not* set off on a quest to discover how Christ performed the miracles of healing that are described in the Bible; nor did he attend the University of Chicago. They can find no evidence. These details, which make Mikao Usui more appealing to a Western and primarily Christian audience, are not supported by any official records.

However, the twenty-one-day fast, meditation, and prayer vigil on Mount Kurama, which culminated in Usui's enlightenment and empowerment to perform healing, and which Takata recognized as the turning point of his life, is also regarded as such by the author of the Usui Memorial in Japan. And the first "miracle of healing" mentioned in Takata's story, Usui's treatment of his own bloodied, stubbed toe, is also considered by the members of today's Usui Reiki Ryoho Gakkai as his first practice of Reiki.

There may be other details that tally when the Usui Shiki Ryoho and Usui Reiki Ryoho accounts are compared more closely. Although Mr. Doi and Rev. Inamoto have rejected a few specific elements of Takata's story of Reiki as inaccurate, the most significant elements are the same—and this is important to remember. Her story still has value—and not only as a matter of historical record. For this reason, the story is still provided in this revised edition, along with some further commentary (see appendix 1).

Yet we may wonder why Takata "embroidered" the truth. Why did she assign Mikao Usui the role of a teacher of religion fascinated by Christ's miracles of healing? Why did she include in her account mention of a trip to consult scholars at the University of Chicago's Department of Religion? She may have wished to please her audience and to make Mikao Usui seem more interesting and likeable to her listeners. If this was her motivation, she acted in keeping with her own heritage and common storytelling practice in Asian cultures, which had no concept of intellectual property or copyright until the late twentieth century. Or she may have deliberately westernized the story to protect Reiki during and after World War II, through a time of strongly anti-Japanese public sentiment. She may also have felt "guided," that is, directed by some inner wisdom, to alter the story slightly—and listened to this guidance because she had found it of value in her own journey to Reiki and in her subsequent practice. It is also possible that all of these factors contributed to her decision to shape the story of Reiki as she did. Undoubtedly, as a result of her decision, Reiki has traveled more easily around the world and been accepted more readily by people of diverse cultures and differing religious beliefs.

Takata characterized Mikao Usui as a hero who does not have all the answers. Instead, he listens attentively; he searches with an open mind; he allows a spiritual question to shape his life into a quest; he perseveres for many years in hope of finding an answer; he is patient, dedicated, and serious in his pursuit of knowledge and wisdom, and finally, he is willing to meditate and to pray for guidance. Takata's story offers comfort to the many people who come to Reiki after long years of searching for healing and for spiritual truth—and it may offer some inspiration and encouragement to those of us today who would like all the answers to our questions about the origin of Reiki already laid out clearly; for now, we must accept that they are not.

We do not find the "truth" of Reiki in its history. Instead, we find it in the experience of the Reiki energy itself, when something in our souls is touched during attunements; and when we feel the flow of healing through our hands and witness muscles relax and pain leave; and when we notice that our lives, day after day, year after year, are transformed by Reiki practice. Old hurts heal and bad relationships dissolve, as our sense of well-being soars, our hearts open to joy, and we accept peace.

Can we even come close to the "truth" of Reiki through attention to its history? It seems unlikely. In the course of a single day of doing research for this revised edition, I found discrepancies in authoritative texts for the year of Mikao Usui's birth, for the year of Hayashi's death, and for the year my own teacher was certified for basic and advanced Reiki—all presented by highly creditable sources, well-known researchers and translators, and students close to the source. One of the reasons for this is that the historical record is incomplete; another is that it is not always consistent.

For the period of time being considered, beginning about a hundred and fifty years ago in rural Japan, few records still exist. How likely is it that any researcher could uncover complete documentation—a paper trail—for Mikao Usui's schooling or his employment or for his travels? Realistically, the chances are slim to none. We know very little about his life from 1865 to the early 1920s; most of the information we have about him spans only the last few years of his life, from his experiences on Mount Kurama to his death in 1926.

What did he tell his students? Although we might hope that his teaching methods and techniques were presented consistently, Mr. Doi tells us, on behalf of the Gakkai, that they evolved over time. As for Mikao Usui's personal history up until his experience on Mount Kurama, he seems to have shared little. Even were he inclined to relate stories of his personal life, he is likely to have told such anecdotes selectively. The same may be said of Dr. Chujiro Hayashi and Mrs. Hawayo Takata. This means that there is not only evidence of evolution in the teaching methods of all three, but there are also discrepancies between accounts of their lives that may not be due to inaccurate record-keeping or fallible memory, but to the teacher's free will and opportunity.

So much, too, is based on interpretation of facts, rather than the facts themselves. For example, Frank Arjava Petter in *The Hayashi Reiki Manual* shares Tadao Yamaguchi's second-hand account of Mrs. Takata's visit to Japan to attend an annual memorial service for Dr. Hayashi: "One person remembers that at the memorial service for Hayashi Sensei in 1952, a lady called Mrs. Takata came from Hawaii to pay her respects. Chie Hayashi Sensei [Dr. Hayashi's widow] asked her to come to Japan permanently and to take over Hayashi Reiki Kenkyu-kai but she declined. It had been too long since she had learned Reiki from Hayashi Sensei and she had already started to alter and popularize it in Hawaii."[8]

Now consider this account of the same event by Helen Haberly, author of *Reiki: Hawayo Takata's Story* and one of Takata's students: ". . . it was several years after the war before Mrs. Takata returned to Tokyo for a visit. She found Mrs. Hayashi in the same place, but great changes had occurred. This was the only building in the area which was untouched by devastation . . ."[9] Mrs. Hayashi had converted the clinic space into living quarters for herself and some orphaned girls and had not continued "the Reiki work'"; Takata ". . . formally returned the property to Mrs. Hayashi, telling her not to shed any more tears over it, as she would go back to Hawaii and spread Reiki to the world from the center there."[10]

While both accounts agree that Takata visited Tokyo to honor her teacher's memory and to pay her respects to Mrs. Hayashi, and that she declined Mrs. Hayashi's invitation to take over Dr. Hayashi's Reiki clinic and institute, the Hayashi Reiki Kenkyu-kai, consider how differently these facts are presented. Which is the truth? This is an issue that occurs again and again when we attempt to reconcile disparities between historical accounts. We must keep an open mind; evaluate what is stated carefully, looking for evidence of unbiased objectivity and scholarly integrity; and yet be guided by our own inner wisdom.

While I acknowledge and value all forms of traditional Reiki now being taught, I teach, as I have taught, Usui Shiki Reiki Ryoho, the style of Reiki that Takata taught to my teacher. I do know now that Takata "translated" Hayashi's teachings into English, dropping Japanese language terms; that she modified the story of Mikao Usui he told to her, at least slightly; and that she evolved her teaching method, changing and simplifying hand positions, developing new distant-healing methods, as she felt guided and appropriate. I also value historical scholarship, so it is without apology that I now offer this updated and revised edition, incorporating the information that has recently been made available through research efforts, translations, and good will and retaining the practical core of instruction that structures any basic course in traditional Western Reiki. I appreciate this moment as an opportunity for healing across cultures and across generations—and I know that such healing is possible, with an open mind, a compassionate heart, and Reiki.

FORWARD TO THE FUTURE

Like many people, I became interested in learning about healing at the bedside of someone I loved whose pain I could not relieve. While I know that my caring and concern, and my prayers, brought some comfort, I still felt frustrated that I could do so little to bring about a positive change. Perhaps as an antidote to relieve my own suffering in this situation, the idea came to me with increasing conviction that such pain as I saw was unnecessary and that a solution to the problem of pain, in harmony with our spiritual natures, was close at hand.

More than a quarter-century later, still pursuing this interest in healing, I decided to take a break from my studies to attend a holistic health conference at Rosemont College in the western suburbs of Philadelphia. I felt contented to spend a day wandering from one fair booth to another, but when I saw that a lecture on Native American medicine would be presented in the early afternoon, I circled it on my program and waited eagerly for it to begin. The lecture turned out to be unimpressive. Not much that was said was new to me. However, as the audience was leaving, I approached a woman who had asked an insightful question and introduced myself. She told me that her name was Angela, and not only was she very interested in Native American medicine, but she also had a Reiki practice.

"Do you know what Reiki is?" she asked.

I didn't, but as soon as she spoke the word, I knew I wanted to learn everything I could about it. When she invited me to make an appointment with her for a Reiki treatment in order to experience it firsthand, I immediately agreed.

Three weeks later I kept my appointment for a Reiki treatment at Angela's house. Her treatment room, which she had converted from a child's bedroom, was now painted with the soothing colors of the desert. The walls were decorated with sandpaintings. She asked if I wanted background music. I opted for quiet and a little conversation.

Angela left the room to allow me to make myself comfortable on her treatment table. I loosened a button at my waist, took off my glasses, lay down on my back, and pulled up the sheet over my pants and flannel shirt.

When she returned, she asked me if I wanted a bolster under my knees, or a blanket for warmth. When I told her I was quite comfortable, she asked permission to begin the treatment and told me she would place her hands first over the bottom of my rib cage (over my flannel shirt and the sheet) and rest them in this position until she felt the energy shift in her hands, which would signal her to move on.

Angela spent perhaps five minutes in this first position. Beneath her hands I could feel a soft, soothing flow of energy. It was nothing startling, but it was relaxing enough that I began to want to nod off. With my conscious mind, however, I resisted the impulse to sleep. I wanted to ask questions.

What did she feel in her hands? I wanted to know. How did she know when to move her hands to the next position? If I felt tingling under her hands, did she feel tingling as well? Could she see my aura? Was she getting any impressions about my health as she worked on me? Angela good-naturedly fielded my questions and continued to give me a full Reiki treatment. Clearly she could engage in conversation without any compromise in the quality of the treatment experience. Apparently she did not need to concentrate or focus her conscious attention on the treatment for the energy to flow through her hands.

With my physical body relaxing and my mind reassured, I asked the most important question of all: When and where could I learn how to do Reiki myself? Angela told me that a Reiki master named Beth Gray was coming to the area in March 1987. I could sign up to take a class with her.

I was frustrated to know that I would have to wait, but glad to have the class to anticipate. As Angela finished the treatment on the front of my body and moved around to work on my head, she told me that she was seeing images in her mind's eye. Although I was unable to interpret some of the images and appreciate their meaning in my life, others were obvious enough to make me laugh. Angela told me that enhanced psychic perception and awareness of past-life experience could also be a product of learning Reiki.

"I want to learn," I thought. "I'm ready for this."

Although I felt ready, it was six months before I was able to take a level I class with Reiki Master Beth Gray and learn the same hands-on method of healing that Angela had demonstrated to me. Daily practice continued to unfold the lessons of this class and strengthened my awareness of the powerful, marvelous energy that now flowed through my hands. The heartfelt surprise and the genuine gratitude for relief from pain of those who unexpectedly benefited from this energy gradually relieved me of all residues of intellectual skepticism.

I began to feel confident that miracles of healing might indeed be possible if only I could put my hands everywhere I saw a need. I pictured my hands inside greater hands than mine that gloved them in a force field of love; for indeed, the feeling of the healing energy surging through my hands did not stop at the boundary of my skin. My hands felt haloed in healing energy. I couldn't wait—and I had to wait—to learn more.

Six months later, in September 1987, I was able to take a level II class with Reiki Master Beth Gray and learn how to send healing at a distance. Again, my awareness of this force field of love shifted and expanded, and my sensitivity to the energy's range of expression significantly increased. Now, as I sent healing at a distance, I had a sense of seeing into the body beneath my hands that reinforced other impressions I was receiving. I shared this information, as appropriate, with the client I worked on, not as prognosis, diagnosis, or prescription, but as impressions and suggestions that were to be consciously and impartially evaluated and used only if deemed meaningful and of benefit.

In the years that followed I returned to assist at level I and II classes every time my teacher came to town—roughly every six months. Every time I returned, I came with questions that had emerged in the course of practicing Reiki. I loved my teacher and believed that every word she spoke was inspired.

The first inkling I had that she was still quite human and capable of growing in her understanding of Reiki occurred when a question I had asked was asked again, six months later, by another student; he received an entirely different answer. The answer she gave this student gives my life purpose and guides my daily practice now.

The question is this: Can we use Reiki to send healing to the world? When I first asked the question at a level II Reiki class at which I was assisting, Beth had just told the new students that they could use the distant-healing method to send Reiki energy not only to people, pets, and plants, but to organizations, to relationships, and to projects—anywhere there was a perceived need. Yet my question surprised her. She hesitated in answering it; then she advised me—and all of us in the room at the time—that it would be better to send healing to individuals, one by one, or to small groups. This answer didn't sit right in the context of what she had just said. I didn't realize it at the time, but I had stumbled onto unmapped territory for her, lessons her teacher, Reiki Master Hawayo Takata, had perhaps not addressed in Beth's presence.

Six months later, when a young man raised his hand and asked the same question at another level II class, I was astonished by Beth's answer. "Can you send Reiki healing to the world?" she said, repeating the question. Then she slowly nodded. "I don't see why not. Try it." Clearly, my Reiki master was capable of opening her mind to new possibilities and adapting to the changing needs of her students.

Five or six years later, when I began to wrestle with my dream of teaching Reiki to others, this understanding of Beth's capacity to change and grow as a human being while serving others as a spiritual teacher helped me see that I might also serve, however unworthy I felt. Now I know that my own humanity is, at times, reassuring to my students, who are concerned with their "readiness" to learn and to practice Reiki at all levels. I am able to regale them with stories of my own lack of readiness—my skepticism, my resistance, my endless questions—and, through the stories, reveal the power of the energy to heal a "doubting Thomas."

I am also able to reassure my students of the value of patience. After I learned Reiki in 1987, eight years passed before I became a teacher. That long interval of time allowed me to practice Reiki; to develop a foundation of experience from this practice; to assist, again and again, at Beth Gray's Reiki classes, in a kind of informal apprenticeship; to grow spiritually; and to develop counseling skills and classroom experience through my other work.

Yet I might not have left the classroom were it not for a dream that woke me from sleep with a haunting sense of urgency in September 1994: I dreamed that a nuclear war had just begun. Everyone had been given fifteen minutes' warning—to evacuate, to get to a bomb shelter, to make peace with themselves and prepare for death. What did I want to do in that time? I wanted to teach Reiki. I watched my dream-self, with fifteen minutes left to live, stop people who were fleeing and begin to talk about hand positions and the flow of energy and Reiki's power of healing.

That morning's realization spurred me to contact by phone one Reiki master after another until I found one with whom I felt an immediate connection and an extraordinary level of trust: I remembered Frank DuGan, a fellow student of Beth Gray's, as someone she had affectionately termed "the Reiki cop"; yet in the years since Beth's retirement, Frank had left the police force to focus on building a Reiki practice and recently had become a Reiki master. I felt a bit intimidated by him, at first: a man who had wedded a lifetime of murder and missing person investigations to the most mystical, joyful experience I knew without missing a beat.

Frank turned out to be the perfect teacher for me: direct to the point of brusqueness, with an investigative mind now focused on the world's spiritual and healing practices, and eyes full of white light. His open mind fostered courage in me to explore what I had accepted through Beth's traditional presentation as the totality of Reiki. He bridged my awareness with a sense of new possibilities and directions.

The perception this has created is still unfolding, of course, but it is marked by an acceptance of the power of Reiki to manifest through many methods, many symbols, many hands. There is no room for self-righteousness in this newly redrawn scheme of the history of Reiki in the world; there can only be tolerance for all the variations already taught and still emerging—and, finally, perhaps, gratitude and appreciation for the immense range of tools that are now at hand for bringing healing to those we love and to the world itself.

This book is written with an eye to a future in which everyone joins hands to bring healing to all those in need and to the earth itself. It is written for those who have never heard of Reiki and for those who use the word in everyday conversation. It is written for those who would like to bring healing to their lives and to the lives of their families, but who do not wish to make Reiki an important focus. It is written for those who are doctors, nurses, allied health professionals, and alternative health professionals, who are looking for new ways to improve the quality of care they can offer, as well as for those who have already recognized that energy medicine enhances the effectiveness and eases the side effects of allopathic treatment, making it an excellent choice for complementary care in the twenty-first century.

This book is also written for those who are already practitioners and teachers of Reiki, as a basic reference, a manual, an invitation to further learning—and as a celebration of the universal life-force energy that flows through our hands. May we reach out to one another in unconditional love to create community, to share visions, and to bring healing to our world.

1

A HEALING METHOD "FOR THE GOOD OF HUMANKIND"

Reiki is a method of natural healing that uses energy channeled through a practitioner's hands to restore health and a sense of well-being. A formal Reiki treatment looks rather like a massage, with two important differences: the client relaxes on the treatment table fully, comfortably clothed; and the practitioner's hands on the client are usually still; the practitioner moves them only when there is a noticeable shift in the flow of channeled energy.

Because the Reiki practitioner's hands remain in position, as the practitioner attends to sensations of a steady energy flow (which may continue for five or ten or twenty minutes unchanged), Reiki treatment is also sometimes compared to laying on of hands. The touch of a Reiki practitioner, like that of a lay healer, is light, gentle, and quiet. However, Reiki is not "faith healing." No

---

The phrase "for the good of humankind" is from Mikao Usui's explanation of Reiki healing in the manual he created for his beginning students, the *Reiki Ryoho Hikkei* (often simply referred to as the Hikkei) or *Reiki Ryoho Handbook*. The manual is called the *Reiki Ryoho no Shiori* by the Usui Reiki Ryoho Gakkai.[1]

faith in the effectiveness of Reiki treatment is required on the part of either the client or the Reiki practitioner. Healing, very simply, occurs.

Even harsh skepticism is no barrier to the healing energy; even a client who lays down on the treatment table saying, "I know this is not going to help me," cannot shut out the healing energy. Why? *Reiki* means "Spirit-guided" or "soul-guided" "life-force." This is a force the conscious mind cannot long resist, for the whole person recognizes its powerful, gentle, loving nature.

The name Reiki is usually translated from Japanese into English as "universal life-force energy." Reiki uses this universal life-force energy, rather than an individual's personal energy, to bring healing to the whole person. It does this in harmony with the natural intelligence of the mind and body, which work together to preserve and protect health and increase well-being.

If, as you read the above paragraphs, you encountered the name Reiki for the first time, you may have been struck by its similarity to some other Asian words that have made their way into our culture. For example, *aikido,* the word for a Japanese martial art, has *ki* at its center. Similarly, *qigong,* a system of Oriental healing and meditation practices, has the word *qi* at its beginning. *T'ai chi,* a form of physical exercise and moving meditation, also has the same word at its root. Whether spelled *ki, qi,* or *chi,* this word refers to life-force energy. These three Asian arts involve cultivating and training one's individual life-force energy for the purpose of self-defense, healing, or meditation.

Reiki differs from these arts in that it does not involve training one's individual life-force energy. Reiki augments the life-force energy that naturally circulates throughout a person's body, sustaining health and vitality, with a strong, powerful flow of the same energy that originally sparks and sets the miracle of life into motion. This energy accelerates and enhances all naturally occurring healing processes: it relaxes tense muscles, speeds digestion, stabilizes blood pressure and blood sugar, stanches the flow of blood, calms a racing pulse, stimulates the immune system, and relieves pain. This makes Reiki an excellent form of preventive medicine for those who are essentially healthy.

For those who face an acute health crisis, such as a cold or the flu or food poisoning, Reiki helps the body to more quickly process the residue of infection and other toxins. Sometimes this simply shortens the duration or diminishes the intensity of symptoms accompanying the crisis; at other times it enables the person to avoid the illness altogether.

Reiki also helps those who are chronically ill to regain a sense of well-being; it alleviates symptoms to such an extent that it often initiates and helps to sustain periods of complete symptom remission. For this reason, when doctors do follow-up tests on patients who have been regularly receiving Reiki treatments as a complement to conventional medical care, they sometimes discover that they can reverse dire diagnoses and change pessimistic prognoses for the better.

Reiki creates and directs healing to those areas of the whole person that can benefit from it. This means that someone who is critically ill can receive healing in areas of the body not yet recognized as diseased by the attending physician (who relies primarily on X-rays and other tests to guide treatment efforts). This also means that the same person, facing a life-or-death health crisis, can often be helped to reclaim the will to live. When a disease or medical condition has already progressed to the point where physical recovery is not possible, Reiki still relieves symptoms, reduces pain, and eases emotional distress; and, at the appropriate time, Reiki assists the whole person in accepting the peace of death.

Not surprisingly, Reiki fosters fertility, and, when a child is conceived, Reiki alleviates the discomforts of pregnancy and eases the pain of childbirth. Sometimes the duration of labor is shortened; sometimes the sensations of discomfort are reduced.

Always, Reiki is healing. Always, Reiki enhances the quality of life, whether the days of life to be lived are many or few. Certainly, when the recipient of a Reiki treatment is chronically or critically ill, the degree of healing that occurs often surprises family members and friends and attending physicians, and even surpasses the expectations of the experienced Reiki practitioner. When the recipient of a Reiki treatment is basically well, however, the healing that occurs does not seem dramatic. Unless very sensitive to energy flow, the healthy client usually only feels more relaxed and in a better mood; this is the consciously accessible correlate of subtle healing.

Whether dramatic or subtle, the experience of healing is not directed by the Reiki practitioner's conscious mind. It is created by the universal life-force energy that flows through the practitioner's hands, in harmony with the life-force that circulates through the mind and body of the individual receiving treatment. The Reiki practitioner simply serves as a channel.

REIKI: A METHOD OF CHANNELING HEALING ENERGY

A Reiki practitioner channels universal life-force energy for the purpose of healing, usually through the palms of the hands. In addition, according to Mikao Usui, Reiki's founder, practitioners can radiate Reiki healing not only through the hands but through "any part of the physical body"[2]; the soft gaze or gentle breath of a practitioner who cultivates awareness of Reiki's subtle energy can be as healing as the touch of Reiki-charged hands.

This ability to channel universal life-force energy sets Reiki apart from both ancient healing traditions and other modern modalities. For example, Reiki differs from "laying on of hands," with which it is often compared, in that it does not require either the "healer" or the recipient of healing to have faith of any kind. People of all religions, as well as agnostics and atheists, can and do learn Reiki and practice it effectively on their clients; people of all religions, as well as agnostics and atheists, can and do receive Reiki treatments and experience wonderful healing benefits. Reiki simply works, on believers and non-believers alike.

Reiki is also unlike shamanism, which has been practiced for thousands of years in tribal cultures. This ancient, honorable tradition requires the healer to take on the sickness of the person in need of healing in order for that person to become free of illness. Reiki does not require taking on anyone else's physical sickness, mental anguish, or emotional suffering. Instead, both the Reiki practitioner and the client receive some healing, although the client who is the intended recipient experiences by far the greatest healing effects.

Reiki is also distinct from some modern healing modalities, such as Swedish massage, which require the practitioner to work the client's tense muscles into a more relaxed state. Reiki does not physically tax or exhaust a practitioner, because no physical effort, other than placing the hands in position, is needed to channel the healing energy. Yet many clients will comment, at the end of a

Reiki treatment, "That was better than a massage." They have felt the soothing effects of the energy so deeply that they dozed off and then awoke completely relaxed and refreshed. Indeed, massage therapists and physical therapists often learn Reiki so that they can offer their clients a healing modality that does not, over time, stress their own muscles and tendons to the point of carpal tunnel syndrome. More and more accredited massage schools offer Reiki among their course listings.

Because the Reiki method of natural healing uses channeled energy of a higher power, the practitioner's energies are not drained. In fact, most Reiki practitioners claim that doing a treatment makes them feel "charged up." This is a product of the flow of the energy itself. It flows into the practitioner first, to bring healing and relief to any area of stress in the practitioner's body, and then it flows through the practitioner's hands to the client. Like the inside of a garden hose, which remains flexible and in good condition when it is used often to water thirsty ground, the practitioner benefits from the flow of energy that courses into her and through her.

Many people feel that the hands they bring to Reiki are already "healing hands." Massage therapists, nurses, doctors, chiropractors—indeed, anyone— can consciously work with imagery, affirmation, and intention to strengthen the healing character of their hands. Reiki greatly enhances whatever natural or cultivated healing ability a student has; if the student feels he has no natural healing ability, Reiki establishes beyond any doubt that the student has been endowed with the ability to channel a higher order of healing power.

The only physical effort that the individual Reiki practitioner needs to make is to put his hands somewhere—on himself, on a client on the treatment table, around a terracotta pot holding a lemon-scented geranium—and the healing energy will flow of its own accord. As long as the Reiki practitioner has been properly attuned to channel the healing energy, then he need not be centered or grounded or spiritually uplifted or even in a good mood. As soon as he puts his hands down, the Reiki energy will flow—and the experience of channeling this healing energy will center and ground and uplift and bring healing to the Reiki practitioner, as well as to the person, the animal, the plant under his hands.

This is one of the great benefits of learning traditional Usui Reiki: by merely cooperating with the energy flow, the practitioner helps to bring about his own healing. This is one of the reasons that Reiki practitioners do not call them- selves "healers." They are well aware that the universal life-force energy is the true healer and does all the real work of healing.

REIKI ATTUNEMENT: A TIMELESS RITUAL OF TRANSFORMATION

What allows Reiki to accomplish in its brief class sessions what other Oriental healing arts cannot accomplish with years of dedicated training? The answer is both simple and profound: Reiki classes include attunements by a Reiki master (teacher), which empower the student to channel universal life-force energy for healing. These attunements are rituals that gently transform the student's aware- ness; they charge the student with universal life-force energy, which aligns the student's individual energy with this higher power and stabilizes the student's ability to channel its strong, healing flow.

Sometimes the attunement experience is a quiet one. Only gradually, some- times weeks or months later, does the student realize the extraordinary trans- formation that has occurred within his hands and his heart. At other times, the attunement experience is quite dramatic. The student reports seeing swirl- ing purple light or a flowering lotus blossom, or hearing the sound of temple gongs. Whether the student perceives no conscious change or is floored by all the bells and whistles makes no difference: he is transformed, awakened into a new way of being whose very nature is healing. As he practices Reiki on himself and others, his awareness will grow stronger. His skepticism will be replaced by faith, and his faith by a profound, intimate, loving knowledge of the healing energy that works through him.

This faith, based on practical experience, is compatible with any religion or spiritual practice. Since Mrs. Hawayo Takata first began teaching Reiki in Hawaii in 1938, many Reiki practitioners have been taught that Reiki is the same healing method used by Christ and the Buddha, rediscovered by a Japanese scholar, Mikao Usui, who dedicated his life to searching for this knowledge. Recent research in Japan and contact with Japanese Reiki practitioners and teachers now makes it possible to describe the origins of Reiki with more accuracy.

In his sixth decade, Mikao Usui, a Pure Land Buddhist, sought to experience enlightenment. He committed himself to a twenty-one day fast, meditation, and prayer vigil on Mount Kurama, a sacred mountain on the outskirts of Kyoto, in hope of achieving a spiritual awakening—or at the very least a peaceful death. At dawn of the twenty-first day, he "suddenly felt the great Reiki energy at the top of his head."*[3] This experience of universal life-force energy completely healed him and radically transformed him so that he could heal himself and others and teach healing as well.

In the manual that he created for his beginner students, the *Reiki Ryoho Hikkei,* Mikao Usui responds to a question about why and how Reiki works: "I have not been taught this art of healing by anyone under the heavens, nor have I studied in order to obtain this mysterious ability to heal. I accidentally realized that I was given this mysterious healing ability when I felt the great power and was inspired by the mystery during a period of fasting. Therefore, even as the founder, I find it difficult to give a sure explanation."[4]

Asked if it is necessary to believe in the effectiveness of Reiki in order for it to work, he answers no and observes, "Barely one out of ten people trust and esteem my art of healing before they experience it the first time. Most people come to trust suddenly after having received treatment once and acknowledged its effect."[5]

Yet he does acknowledge that the source of "the healing power of the universe" is "heavenly" in nature:

My Usui Reiki Ryoho (healing art) is original, never before explored, and incomparable in the world. Therefore, it is to be made available for the good of humankind, so that anyone may be blessed with this heavenly gift, that the soul and body may be as one, and heaven-sent well-being may be realized in one's life. Because my Reiki Ryoho is a unique and original art of healing based on the healing power of the universe, a person first becomes healthy and then soundness of thought and the joys of life are enhanced.[6]

*This phrase is from the first published translation into English of the inscription on the Usui Memorial, which is located to one side of Mikao Usui's grave in the cemetery outside the Saihoji Temple in the Toyatoma section of Tokyo.

Mikao Usui was referred to as "Dr. Usui" by his contemporaries, who wanted to express their regard for him as a great healer and spiritual teacher, despite his lack of formal training as a physician. He treated countless people and taught approximately 2,000 people* the Reiki method so that they could continue the work of healing themselves and offer healing to others. He ensured that the teaching of Reiki would continue after he left this world. He did not turn Reiki into a religion: he did not set himself above others; he did not write down any commandments; he did not write scripture. In fact, he did not ask anyone to believe anything about Reiki—not even that it works. He encouraged all those who came to him for healing—and they were of various religious persuasions—simply to experience Reiki and to allow it to enhance their quality of life, mind, body, and soul.

In simple truth, Reiki does not conflict with any religion. What Reiki does provide is a direct, profound experience of the healing power of Spirit-guided life-force energy. Some Reiki practitioners feel comfortable regarding this as a direct experience of God and practice Reiki as part of their personal spiritual path. Others, who come to Reiki with no particular religious beliefs, are content to see this as a transforming experience of powerful, healing energy, and do not concern themselves with its ultimate source.

Perhaps in the course of the next one or two hundred years people will turn Reiki into a religion complete with a bureaucratic administration, a "clergy," doctrines, and all the other trappings of orthodoxy. At this point in time, however, there are no good reasons to complicate the process of teaching Reiki or providing Reiki treatments. The simplicity and directness of the experience of feeling healing energy coursing through the hands is profound, humbling, uplifting, and equally available to all. No philosophy, no doctrine, no dogma stands in anyone's way of experiencing this healing energy—and that is as it should be.

"Universal life-force energy" must, to live up to its name, support and sustain the growth and development of every single person, whatever his or her religious beliefs. For Reiki is a practical and effective natural healing method; while the techniques of Reiki practice and the methods of its teaching can be

---

*The author of the Usui Memorial lists this as one of Mikao Usui's achievements; this figure is mentioned in all translations.

traced to early 1920s' Japan, the essence of the energy is beyond chronological time. The use of similar "laying on of hands" healing methods are recorded across ancient scriptures. It is one of the wonders of our time that through Reiki we can learn to connect with the same energy that has flowed through the hands of past spiritual masters without the necessity of spiritual faith. Why? Perhaps the answer is simply that the world needs so much healing.

For this reason, out of the usual context of practices for the purpose of individual spiritual enlightenment, Dr. Usui offered Reiki to the people in his community. He did not require that they give up old beliefs or adopt new ones, nor did he ask them to take up other spiritual disciplines to provide a foundation for the healing they had received. He offered Reiki with no strings attached, although he did encourage them to appreciate and value the healing they received.

Now the world is the community that is offered Reiki through the hands of many Reiki masters and Reiki channels. As we practice Reiki and see it work in our own lives, it stretches our ability to believe in miracles. Reiki offers the greatest hope we know to heal ourselves and our world.

2

REIKI IN THE CONTEXT OF OUR TIME

REIKI'S ORAL—AND WRITTEN—TRADITION

Often, the first Reiki story that a new practitioner tells is of the events in his life that led him to be in the Reiki I class. Perhaps a coworker saw him struggling to ward off a headache and offered to do some healing, or he crossed the finish line at a marathon and encountered a volunteer who smiled and offered Reiki-charged hands to soothe his exhausted body. Whatever prompts a student to learn Reiki, the story of that first encounter with Reiki healing energy is one he is likely to repeat, as he matter-of-factly introduces Reiki to others, now and again, over the course of his life. Should this new practitioner eventually decide to become a teacher, he will find himself telling this story in almost every level I class that he teaches. This story, because it chronicles an important episode in his life journey, will move his audience more than any objective account he gives of Reiki's benefits. Because we continue to learn about Reiki long after class is over, through the experience of the energy channeled for healing during self- and client treatment, we gradually accumulate many memories of our experiences—and when we share our accounts of these experiences through storytelling, we educate others about Reiki.

Here is an example of a story that I sometimes tell in level I Reiki classes, if someone wants to know more about using Reiki in animal healing:

"You said that Reiki can be helpful to pets. How about animals in nature?" a newly attuned student asks.

"Well, when I first began to practice Reiki, I had no pets," I admit. "I love animals, but I lived in an apartment in Philadelphia that had a lease restriction, so I followed the rules. I lived without cats, hamsters, and even goldfish.

"One day, I was sitting at my kitchen table with one of my graduate school textbooks open before me, highlighting passages and taking notes. I felt my hands surge on for no apparent reason. I looked around the kitchen, then out the window beside me. About fifteen feet away, a robin sat on a tree branch staring back at me. So I thought perhaps she needed Reiki. I set down my highlighter and my pen, reoriented my chair for a better view, and then lifted up my hands, so that my palms could radiate Reiki healing to the robin. The draw was surprisingly intense—and the robin stayed on that branch for about fifteen minutes before the energy shifted and she flew away. I think she really did need Reiki—and she came to my window to ask for it."

The students are intrigued.

"You will find that you can 'beam' Reiki energy this way at animals in the wild that need healing, but that won't come near enough to touch. It's very attractive to them. Once when I visited a wilderness refuge, I knelt in the grass beside a pond and radiated the energy through my raised hands to a whole bunch of ducklings. They all turned toward me and started waddling in my direction, much to the surprise of their mothers!"

The students laugh with me. When they quiet down, I continue: "You can also use this technique on people, of course, say when you notice someone who seems to be upset or uncomfortable at another table in a restaurant. You can use the same technique when you drive by the scene of an accident or see an ambulance approaching in the opposite lane. If you are driving, just hold up one hand, and if you are the passenger, use both hands to radiate some Reiki healing to those in need of healing."

One of the students hesitantly lifts her hands, palms outward, in my direction.

"Yes, yes!" I say. "It's that simple. Let's all try it. Just raise your hands up to about chest height, palms facing outward, and direct the energy to the person beside you."

"I can feel that! I can feel my hands tingling," one student says to another.

She is rewarded with a thoughtful smile and a comment: "That's amazing! I can feel myself receiving the energy you're sending all up and down my left side and through my shoulders. That's just where I need it today, too!"

This brief Reiki story has served more than one purpose: it has answered a question, opened up discussion, and led to demonstration of a specific technique. This is an example of how Reiki is often taught in the classroom. Most traditional Reiki masters teaching a level I class, besides attuning new students four times, teaching hand positions for self-treatment and client treatment, and relaying a history of Reiki, will use storytelling to illustrate how the Reiki energy works and how effective it is in providing healing benefits in many different kinds of situations. When we share what we have come to know about Reiki through such stories of our experience, we participate in an "oral tradition" of teaching. (This book, which is meant to be usable as a manual for traditional Reiki masters and also helpful as a reference work for Reiki practitioners after completion of the level I class, is deliberately spare in terms of stories; it is my hope that the practical instruction here will be supplemented with many stories from your Reiki master's own experience.)

How did storytelling come to be so important in teaching Reiki? When Mikao Usui's healing method was first taught and practiced in Japan in the early 1920s, not everyone who was interested in learning Reiki could read. In addition, not everyone could afford to buy books for themselves; a personal library was a luxury.* In a culture that had valued the oral tradition of spiritual teaching for

---

*Japanese Reiki Master Hiroshi Doi has shared anecdotal evidence describing the development of Reiki distant-healing methods, which implies that Mikao Usui taught people without regard to their educational accomplishments, social class, or economic level. Initially, practitioners were invited to use photographs to connect to their clients, but since not many people had photographs available or could afford to have them made, the method soon evolved into "picture Reiki," which required only a drawing of the client, quickly rendered by the practitioner and then destroyed after the treatment was completed. Eventually, practitioners and teachers realized that a physical image is not necessary at all to successfully send distant healing; visualization, used with one of the many Reiki distant-healing techniques, can be sufficient to ensure that the client receives healing.

thousands of years, Dr. Usui found a way to teach his students that relied primarily upon experiential learning. He formed a learning society called the Usui Reiki Ryoho Gakkai, which provided a venue for him to teach his methods in person, meditating with his students, demonstrating techniques, and observing them as they practiced and learned to attend to Reiki's healing flow.

In addition, he supplied a written manual of basic information printed in small booklet form. This manual, called the *Usui Reiki Ryoho Hikkei* or the *Usui Reiki Handbook,* includes a brief table of contents; the Gainen (familiar in abbreviated form to practitioners around the world as the Reiki principles); his explanation of Reiki presented in question-and-answer format; a list of recommended hand positions for treatment of some illnesses and medical conditions; and finally, the Gyosei, a selection of brief, inspirational poems composed by the Meiji Emperor.[1]

Usui gave this manual to his Shoden (beginner) students. (There is no evidence that he created a manual for his Okuden [advanced] or Shinpiden [master] students.) Once he had attuned the Shoden students to the Reiki energy through a brief ceremony, which often included meditation, recitation of the Gainen, and sometimes the reading or singing of a poem, he showed them how to do five simple hand positions on the head. He encouraged the new practitioners to reflect upon the Gainen each morning and night, to practice the Reiki hand positions he had demonstrated on themselves and others, and to consult the manual for help whenever they treated someone suffering from injury or infection, acute or chronic illness, or any serious medical condition. (The manual did not discuss treatment of such conditions at great length, because Usui knew that with practice, these new practitioners would develop increasing sensitivity to the flow of Reiki healing energy, as well as to the subtle imbalances in the body's physical energy. The ability to sense this resonance—called *hibiki*—and to scan the body to detect areas in need of healing treatment—called Byosen-ho—became the criteria for advancement from Shoden to Okuden level. Today's Gakkai still distributes Usui's handbook to new students and uses mastery of these two particular techniques as the criteria for advancement from Shoden to Okuden.)

Mikao Usui treated people with Reiki and taught them how to perform the Reiki method of healing only during the last years of his life, from the time of his own spontaneous attunement to the Reiki energy on Mount Kurama (Mr. Hiroshi Doi dates this event to March 1922, but other accounts place it earlier[2]) until his death on March 9, 1926.[3] While researchers continue to search for letters, diaries, notes, newspaper articles—anything which might offer more insight into Mikao Usui's character or provide a clearer understanding of his practice and teaching methods—the *Usui Reiki Ryoho Hikkei* is the most important text from that time period and it will probably remain so, because it is the only primary source to be identified so far. Mikao Usui himself created this manual: he adopted the five principles from another author,[4] framing them with his own double title and a recommendation to use them in meditation; he wrote the answers to the frequently asked questions; he compiled the list of recommended hand positions for particular ailments; and he selected the inspirational poems that conclude the manual from thousands written by this particular Meiji Emperor. While there are a few important secondary source materials that have now been translated and made available to practitioners and teachers interested in Reiki's early history, the Hikkei is the only written evidence that we have of what Mikao Usui presented to his students and what he wanted them to remember after he concluded his initial instruction.

Reiki teachers from Mikao Usui's time to our own have continued to rely on a strong oral classroom presentation, with lecture, demonstration, question and answer, and sometimes storytelling to teach specific techniques. Dr. Chujiro Hayashi, Hawayo Takata's teacher, like Dr. Usui before him, also created a Hikkei or handbook for his students.* Unlike Dr. Usui's handbook, Dr. Hayashi's focuses completely on the practicalities of Reiki treatment for specific injuries and illnesses, diseases, and chronic conditions. This echoes the classroom content that Hawayo Takata described to biographer Helen J. Haberly:

> During the lessons he explained the treatment, the first day dealing with the body above the neck—the head, eyes, ears, nose, and throat—and the conditions and disease which would be found in these areas. On the second

---

*Frank Arjava Petter offers translations of both of these two important primary sources: *The Original Reiki Handbook of Dr. Mikao Usui* and *The Hayashi Reiki Manual.*[5] Petter's books are supplemented with photographs and illustrations demonstrating the recommended hand positions for various medical conditions; William Rand also provides a translation of Dr. Hayashi's handbook in his *Reiki: The Healing Touch; First and Second Degree Manual.*[6] and John and Lourdes Gray, in *Hand to Hand,*[7] present yet another translation.

day [students] were taught how to treat the front of the body, the chest and abdomen, with all the organs located here. The lesson for the third day dealt with the back, which included the spine, nerve systems, and organs. They were shown where and how to place their hands to permit the Life Energy to flow to the body of the patient, allowing Reiki to balance the condition or ailment so healing could occur.

On the fourth day Dr. Hayashi discussed how to heal in acute cases, such as accidents. He also spoke of the spiritual side of Reiki, for which were given the Five Ideals . . .[8]

Perhaps to emphasize the beauty and grace of the Reiki principles, Dr. Hayashi handwrote them in Japanese *kanji*, had a stamp made from the image, and then imprinted this image onto paper fans, which he gave to some of his students.[9] For his Japanese students, he created certificates in Japanese calligraphy, marked with his chop, or official stamp.[10]

However, for Mrs. Hawayo Takata, who arrived at his clinic in 1935 as a patient and whom he certified in 1938 as a master in the City of Honolulu, Hawaii, Dr. Hayashi created a master certificate in English. He clearly intended that it be a matter of public record that he regarded Takata as well qualified to practice and to teach Reiki. His confidence in her must surely have comforted her as she sought out a property for a center and began her career.

Before Dr. Hayashi's death in May 1940, Takata visited him again. He discussed with her his concern that the coming war between Japan and America might be disruptive to the practice and teaching of Reiki, in his homeland and in hers. He gave her the responsibility of safeguarding Reiki through the turbulent years ahead. Because she revered him as her teacher and because she took very seriously her responsibility to keep Reiki "alive and well" through World War II and its aftermath, she made some difficult choices: she dropped Japanese language terms (she even used "short wave" treatment instead of the word "Reiki" on her signage, at one point[11]); she simplified techniques; and when she taught, she modified the story of Mikao Usui to make him seem more appealing to a Western audience; and she embraced the oral tradition of spiritual teaching. She never made a manual. For years, she even refused to allow her students to take notes. Even with her Reiki master students, she did not allow notes on the symbols* or on the attunement process. They were required to learn by memory, which is both selective and subjective in its interpretation.

During most of Takata's more than forty-year career, from 1938, when Dr. Hayashi placed her master certificate on file in the City of Honolulu, until her death in 1980, she maintained this position. The few writings that we have by her exist in two forms: a few unpublished diary entries that she wrote during her training with Dr. Hayashi and a few published entries, also regarded as "early writing," initially collected by her daughter, Alice Takata Furumoto, in *Reiki: A Memorial to Takata Sensei* in 1982 and later included in *Reiki: The Usui System of Natural Healing* in 1985, by her granddaughter, Phyllis Furumoto.[12]

Yet toward the end of her life, there is some evidence that Takata's viewpoint regarding the importance of the oral tradition of teaching Reiki began to change and to soften. In the February 24, 1974 *Honolulu Advertiser,* Patsy Matsuura, a staff writer, interviewed Mrs. Takata and elicited from her the information that she was "busy writing a book, *Look Younger, Feel Stronger, and a Way to Longevity. . . .*"[13] Although this manuscript may exist somewhere in partial or complete form, it was never published. Also, in a 1975 Reiki I class, she distributed typed handouts and allowed her students to take notes without remarking upon it.[14] And finally, over the course of several visits to Beth and John Gray's home in California during the 1970s, she allowed them to record some of her stories, presented during classes, on audiocassette tape. (These stories, long after Takata's death, were compiled and edited by John and Lourdes Gray onto a single tape called, "Takata Speaks,"[15] which is available to the general public.)

During the course of Takata's long career, like everyone who conscientiously practices Reiki, she continued to learn from her experiences of the Reiki energy and this enabled her to evolve her teaching methods. Perhaps surprisingly, without informing her students, she sometimes taught different techniques for hands-on and distant healing—one way of emphasizing that Reiki, universal life energy, accomplishes the work of healing, rather than one or another "right"

---

*There is one known exception: a page of the symbols, purportedly drawn by Takata, was preserved by Virginia Samdahl, one of her first Reiki master students.

method.* Even the Reiki masters she initiated, who often traveled internationally to teach, taught as they were taught, without being aware that they had been taught differently from one another—and because they taught in relative isolation from one another, few of them ever discovered or discussed these differences.

Perhaps it was inevitable that in an increasingly interconnected world, discovery of Takata's variations in teaching methods and techniques would become inevitable and discussion necessary. When Diane Stein's controversial book, *Essential Reiki: A Complete Guide to an Ancient Healing Art,* was published with illustrations of the Reiki symbols and their variations in 1995,[21] practitioners began to question the Reiki masters who had attuned them, and these masters began to talk more openly with other masters. It became clear that Takata had taught variations in method. Why? Perhaps she was responding to some inner guidance regarding the techniques that would be

---

*To understand how much variation occurred, consider the following: In an early diary entry, published in *Reiki: The Usui System of Natural Healing,* Takata writes: "Start treatment from the eyes, sinus, pituitary glands, ears, throat, thyroids [sic], thymus, stomach, gall bladder, liver, pancreas, solar plexus, ileocecum, colon, sigmoid flexure, ovarian glands, bladder, then front chest and heart. Turn patient over, treat the back, lungs, sympathetic nerves, kidneys, spleen, and prostate gland. During the treatment, trust in your hands".[16]

John and Lourdes Gray, in *Hand to Hand,* say that Takata created a "foundation treatment," which focused "on the torso and the head. Four basic hand positions were for the torso, three positions for the head, and no positions over the heart or on the back. She supplemented her foundation treatment with optional positions, depending on the nature of the client's problem and where it was physically located."[17]

Helen Haberly, in *Reiki: Hawayo Takata's Story,* writes: "Specific hand positions are taught for the sake of expedience since long practice has shown these to work efficiently; however, there is no 'wrong' way to do Reiki—and, thus, no 'right' way." Yet, she notes, Takata ". . . emphasized treating the abdomen, the Foundation Treatment, teaching that most ailments and disharmonies in the body originate here from poorly functioning organs with low vitality."

"In her classes she demonstrated the proper hand positions for complete treatment, and she noted there are three major areas to be considered: the front, especially the abdomen; the head; and the back. . . . The order in which the Reiki is done does not matter, so long as the full treatment is given, but it usually starts with the head or abdomen."[18]

William Lee Rand reports, in an article entitled "Takata's Handouts" in the Summer 2009 issue of *Reiki News Magazine* that Takata listed "Basic positions: 1, 2, 3, 4, in front of the body / 1, 2, 3 in back of body" in her handouts to a 1975 class. There is no mention of treatment of the head.[19]

Takata-trained Reiki Master Virginia Samdahl taught to start with three hand positions on the head, then continue with four on the abdomen, and four on the back, according to *The Reiki Handbook* by Larry Arnold and Sandy Nevius.[20]

Takata-trained Reiki Master Beth Gray, my teacher, on whose basic course this book is based, taught to start with four hand positions on the abdomen, then four on the head, and then four on the back, for self-treatment, and more, to cover the whole length of the back from shoulders to sacrum, on a client.

of most value to each group of students—or perhaps she did so deliberately to preserve the essential truth of Reiki: the energy itself is the healer—and it is also the teacher.

The practice of Reiki offers us the chance to work in cooperation with universal life-force energy. Through practice, we discover that this energy is conscious, purposeful, intelligent, and infinitely loving, as God is conscious, purposeful, intelligent, and infinitely loving. This energy ignores differences in spoken and written language and hand gesture, and is not deflected from its purpose by imprecision, inattention, lack of clear intent, emotional or mental distress, or flaws of character. Its nature is so compassionate that it instantly compensates for our inadequacies. The energy brings healing into the world, and nothing we can say or do can turn it from this purpose, prevent it from accomplishing this end, or diminish its power.

While the oral tradition of teaching Reiki will always be helpful to those who want to learn to be effective practitioners and teachers, the political climate that caused Takata to insist that her students take no notes has changed. The suspicion, fear, and intolerance she must have felt as a Japanese-American in the 1940s and 1950s have healed. Through her long years of vigilance, she succeeded in ensuring that Reiki did more than survive—in fact, because of her efforts and those of the Reiki masters she initiated before her death in 1980, traditional Reiki is now practiced by millions of people worldwide.

Contemporary Reiki masters who regard themselves as traditional make peace with the past in many ways. Most still maintain at least some of what they have been taught—usually the symbols and attunement techniques—as secret, and pass this information to their students solely through reliance on oral transmission. In the classroom setting, however, faced with students who want to learn techniques of hands-on or distant healing and learn them well, most encourage note-taking or provide handouts or brief manuals, as Dr. Usui and Hayashi did for their beginner students. Today's traditional Reiki masters also recognize that knowledge gained through many years of experience of the Reiki energy is a solid foundation for teaching, and it can be the basis for the anecdotes that are most inspiring and meaningful to students. So they tell stories! And they remind their students that they, too, will have their "first miracle,"* and that long after the class is over, their practice of Reiki will continue to teach them about healing, about spirituality, and about the nature of the energy itself.

THE REIKI MASTER

The Reiki master, who will teach you Reiki, is, first and foremost, an individual who has received a master attunement, a much more powerful attunement than that received by students in hands-on and distant-healing classes. This attunement highly charges him with the Reiki energy, healing and bringing up for cleansing whatever remains in his consciousness to be healed and cleansed. This attunement also refines, greatly strengthens, and stabilizes the channel for healing established through earlier attunements. For the new Reiki master must serve as a conduit for stronger flows of energy than he has ever experienced before. Like a lightning rod, he must serve to channel all the energy that any student can accept and assimilate with conscious awareness. The student will "hold" this energy from one attunement to the next, becoming, with each attunement, a stronger, clearer channel.

The amount of energy that a student receives and accepts during an attunement is not in the control of the Reiki master. Just as a client on a treatment table receives the amount of Reiki energy that is exactly right for the body to work with at the time of treatment, so the student in a class receives the amount of energy that is exactly right for the channel for healing to be established at the time of attunement.

The amount of energy that any one student can receive with comfortable awareness during the attunement varies. Sometimes there is no awareness of change at all. Yet the Reiki master will be very aware of the strong energy flowing through his hands and into and through each student being attuned.

This awareness is healing to the Reiki master; it is also awe inspiring. The commitment to serve as a Reiki master, teaching the minds and attuning the hands of students, must be strong in order for the master not to be deflected

---

*Rev. Beth Gray liked to tell her level I students, who were awed by her stories, "You will have your first miracle." I heard this again and again at the Reiki I classes at which I assisted from 1987 to 1993, when she retired from teaching.

from his purpose by a sense of unworthiness. (The Reiki master has his own life lessons, given to help him grow and evolve; he may be selfish, narrow-minded, proud, or judgmental. Whatever the weaknesses of his character, sooner or later he becomes aware of them and learns to accept the importance of his own self-healing.) Continued service rewards the master with greater understanding and experience of the nature of this healing energy, which is unconditional love. With this comprehension comes greater self-acceptance and a renewed desire to serve.

As he teaches, the Reiki master may speak with true inspiration, saying exactly the words that his students need to hear in a voice that has the tones of healing. As he teaches, he may also mispronounce words or stutter, contradict something he said a moment earlier, or admit he does not know the answer to a question. If he does so, be grateful for his honesty in admitting the limits of his experience and intellectual knowledge. He is showing his humanity and his own trust in the energy, as well as demonstrating mastery. When you feel uncertain of your own hands or the evidence of your own experience, this may offer you an insight into faith.

A traditional Reiki master will acknowledge Mikao Usui's experience of spiritual enlightenment and healing empowerment on Mount Kurama as the beginning of "the Usui system of Reiki healing" taught by Hawayo Takata as Usui Shiki Ryoho.* This is the same term most of the Reiki masters she initiated placed on their students' certificates, and it is still used today worldwide by many Reiki masters to indicate their lineage through a Takata-trained Reiki master to Takata, Hayashi, and Usui. If you are taught Reiki in a traditional class modeled on Hawayo Takata's presentation of the system, Usui Shiki Ryoho or Usui Shiki Reiki Ryoho† is very likely to be indicated on the certificate you

---

*When I learned Reiki level III, Frank DuGan told me that Usui Shiki Ryoho could be translated as "the Usui school of natural healing." In *Reiki Fire,* Petter translates this more broadly as "style, form or system," but also uses the phrase *shiki ryoho* to mean "school," as in this sentence: "A little earlier that year, one of our students had given us the phone number of the Usui Shiki Ryoho in Tokyo."[22] Also, Dr. Hayashi uses the term "Usui system of Reiki healing" on the certificate he created for Hawayo Takata to indicate her complete qualification to teach Reiki healing to others.

†In an e-mail dated 4/6/2010, William Rand wrote: "the words Usui Shiki Ryoho mean Usui Method System in Japanese—Shiki and Ryoho mean almost the same thing. One of my Japanese students who lives in Kyoto gave me this information. She says that there is a word missing from this phrase and that to make sense it really should be Usui Shiki Reiki Ryoho which would then mean the Usui Method of Reiki System." While Hawayo Takata wrote "Usui Shiki Ryoho" on the certificates she gave to her students, and they, in turn, gave to the next generation of students they initiated, "Usui Shiki Reiki Ryoho" has become more widely accepted.

receive at the completion of your class as well, as part of the printed or written text of the document and as part of the Reiki master's seal.

THE REIKI CLASS

Traditional Reiki (sometimes called Usui Shiki Ryoho or Western Reiki) is taught worldwide in three levels. The first level (level I) teaches the student hands-on healing; the second level (level II) teaches the student distant healing; the third level (level III) trains the experienced Reiki practitioner to teach Reiki.

During a level I class, a traditional Reiki master is required to present a history of Reiki; to demonstrate the hands-on healing positions the student should use to treat himself; to demonstrate the hands-on healing positions the student should use to treat a client; and to provide four attunements to establish the student as a channel for healing. This is the instructional "core" of a level I class. Once these requirements are met, the Reiki master provides a level I certificate to the student to document completion of the training and qualification to set up a professional Reiki practice.

However, other components may be added to the teaching curriculum to complement this instructional core. Silent prayer, guided meditation, and question-and-answer sessions are common additions. Discussion of the intimate relationship between the mind and the body is considered by many Reiki masters to be important. Capping off the class with individual student practice providing a complete Reiki treatment to a client on the treatment table is beneficial, particularly for those students who are already bodyworkers and who will add Reiki to the list of alternative healing services they offer.

There is no need, however, in a Reiki level I class, to make other alternative healing methods, such as chakra balancing, aura cleansing, and polarity, a strong focus of discussion. The Reiki master's task is to teach Reiki. Her time is best spent making sure that all the students feel the Reiki energy flow in their hands and are confident of the subtle shifts in the energy that signal that it is time to move to another hand position, rather than providing instruction in other alternative healing methods readily available elsewhere.

The Reiki level I class, after all, is a meeting of minds, many for the first time. Although our culture shows evidence of increasing interest in alternative healing methods, not everyone who is interested in learning Reiki wants to do so in a room that has been smudged with cedar or made smoky with incense. Although Reiki may be the culmination of one student's extensive exploration of alternative healing, for another student it may be the first step. For this reason, diluting discussion of Reiki with details of such explorations by a single student or even by the Reiki master can diminish the experience of the class for those who wish simply to learn Reiki.

For some students it is everything they can do to sit through the class, calming self-doubt and skepticism long enough to listen to the Reiki master's instruction and to their hands. Still, they are ready to learn Reiki or they would not be there. For these students, a Reiki master who clearly focuses on the simplicity of Reiki offers essential support.

THE REIKI STUDENT

In more than twenty years of practicing Reiki, most of the people I have seen learn Reiki have been householders, people who work in jobs that have nothing in particular to do with healing, but who have a desire to be able to give healing to their children, spouse, or an ailing relative. Initially, only a few people in each class were already involved in healing—as physicians, nurses, chiropractors, physical therapists, massage therapists, and so on—but since the mid-1990s, the number of health and allied health professionals learning Reiki has risen dramatically. Many of these health professionals decide to learn Reiki because this alternative healing method will help them move forward professionally.

For example, registered nurses in every state can apply for continuing education units for completing a Reiki I class taught by a qualified professional. Massage therapists at some state-certified schools are offered Reiki as an elective, as part of their five- or six-hundred hour course of training. Some take a Reiki class not for credit, but simply to improve the quality of their patient care. This makes both alternative and traditional health-care professionals more employable in hospitals, hospices, clinics, physicians' and chiropractors' offices, and even spas.

Finally, some people decide to learn Reiki to help them make a transition "out of the rat race" and into a more satisfying profession and healthier lifestyle. When people make the decision to learn Reiki with this in mind, some wonderful results can be created. A novelist is on call to her veterinarian for emergency-care assistance. An enthusiastic gardener now has a growing business selling Reiki-energized seeds. Some practitioners record original music on cassettes to provide relaxing background sounds for client treatments. Such creative expressions of individual talents and skills can be expected to occur in the life of any Reiki practitioner who wants to make a positive career change. Although the development of unique home businesses does take time, the flow of Reiki energy through the hands as a person sets to work clarifying and setting goals enhances the sense of possibilities and can accelerate the process of achievement.

Of the students who attend a Reiki class, a few are conscious of being on a spiritual path and see Reiki as a natural next step. Then there are those who stumble upon Reiki as if it were a stone in their way; they pick it up and pocket it without knowing why. Only later do they realize that they have culled a rough diamond from the crust of the earth.

Any occupation and any level of awareness of alternative healing methods can provide a foundation of understanding for a student to learn Reiki. Sometimes, however, people are clearly not ready. They respond to being offered a Reiki treatment by brushing aside the practitioner's hand. They interrupt the story a practitioner is telling or simply refuse to listen and walk away.

A young woman who came for a Reiki treatment because she was considering taking a level I class was awed by what occurred during her treatment. She felt well, rested, peaceful, and as though she had experienced a healing force that came from God. She did not feel worthy of such transformation. She left the treatment room saying, "I feel wonderful, but I don't feel ready to learn this."

Such self-judgment can be an obstacle; superstition and fear can also form a block; the pride of ego, when identity is threatened, can create resistance. For this reason, readiness is all. When the sense of unworthiness diminishes, when self-doubt is set aside, when the worry about what others may think is put in perspective, then the student who decides he is ready to learn Reiki will discover that the universe supports his decision in many serendipitous ways.

Yet it is important to understand that even a student who says, "Yes, I am ready to learn Reiki," may not feel entirely ready. There is, after all, no requirement that the student come to Reiki believing that it works; experience teaches this so quickly that belief is not essential. A healthy skepticism, which tests the teacher with question after question, is a good sign of serious interest and commitment. There is room for many a "doubting Thomas" in every Reiki class—scientists who use the empirical method to check their results every day, academics who are trained to intellectual rigor, and those who live by the common-sense philosophy of "Show me. I'm from Missouri."

Still, you will know when you are ready to learn Reiki. You will find yourself parked in the middle of a bookstore aisle, browsing through the pages of a book about Reiki. You will be offered a Reiki treatment for a headache or a backache and love the way it quickly relieves your pain. You will see an article about a teacher who is offering a Reiki class that you can conveniently attend. Or you will call a phone number at the bottom of an advertisement about a Reiki class and find you are connected instantly to someone whose gentle honesty and warmth are immediately attractive and whose answers to your questions indicate that the class will provide you with the kind of environment for learning that you would like. Everything will fall into place. The universe will support you in all your commitments to growth, creativity, and healing.

Reiki Level I

Because the Reiki energy is the true teacher and, through the attunement process, transforms each person who attends a Reiki class as a student into a practitioner equipped to channel healing energy, Reiki cannot be learned by reading a book. However, the concepts regarding healing that are presented through lecture, the methods of practice demonstrated at the bodywork table, and the general content of the discussions that occur when a question is raised and answered can be shared without detracting, in any way, from the Reiki energy.

What follows is typical of the lectures and discussions that occur in a traditional Usui Reiki level I class; "typical," however, does not mean "textbook guided." Although a traditional Reiki master will provide four attunements, teach hand positions for self-treatment and client treatment, and tell a history of Reiki, the attunements, hand positions, and history may vary from those described here. The Reiki master is usually simply following the standard set by his own teacher; as long as he attunes you properly, the Reiki energy will flow. Experiences with Reiki practice will teach you the rest.

3

BASICS OF PRACTICE

DISCOVERING COMMON GROUND

Most Reiki classes begin with a few moments of introduction. The Reiki master will introduce herself and perhaps tell how she came to learn Reiki. She will also ask the students in the classroom to say their names and to talk a little about themselves and what has brought them to this class.

> *"The class was advertised on a flyer in a community center. I knew as soon as I saw the name that I wanted to learn. So I signed up, even though I don't know anything about it."*
>
> *"A friend of mine did some Reiki on me in the office one day on our lunch hour. I had a headache and she asked if she could put her hands on my head and try to do a little massage or something. I told her to go right ahead, because the headache was so bad that I couldn't even eat my lunch. So she put her hands on my head—one on my forehead and one on the back of my head—and that was all she did. She didn't move her hands. And my headache went away in a couple of minutes! After that I asked her what she was doing, and she told me. I knew I wanted to learn."*
>
> *"My sister sent me a distant healing from Argentina, and the results were so positive that I decided that I had to learn."*
>
> *"This man in my aikido class saw me take a bad fall and sprain my ankle. After the first-aid kit was done with, he came up to me and offered to do some healing*

33

over the Ace bandage. I told him to go ahead and do it, because it really hurt. And the pain went away. And then it healed really fast. I was impressed."

"I'm a registered nurse, and I work in the emergency room. I usually work night shifts. Sometimes I work double shifts. I always do overtime. I heard about this book by an emergency room doctor who uses Reiki on some of her patients, and she really helps them. So I tried to find the book because I wanted to read her case notes, but I couldn't find it. Then I saw this announcement about this class this weekend, and I realized that I actually had off for the first time in two months. That was too much of a coincidence. I signed up for the class."

"Well, I don't have anything going on in my life like that, but I heard that Reiki can help you grow spiritually. So I looked for a class, and here I am."

The very first class that I taught had four students in it—a married couple who wanted help coping with the woman's multiple sclerosis, a massage therapist, and a university student who had emigrated to the United States from Russia and had relatives still living near Chernobyl. These people from quite diverse backgrounds discovered they had much to share, for they had a common purpose: to learn the Reiki method of healing.

This manages to connect people who might otherwise never even meet. They discover that it is easy to talk to their classmates. They find that it is easy to make new friends. Nothing dissolves the differences between people like Reiki energy, which is really the energy of unconditional love.

Sometimes the students attending a Reiki class have come on impulse or on someone's advice; they might never have felt the sensations of energy that accompany the application of Reiki hands. If the size of the class allows, I invite such students to experience the Reiki energy on the treatment table. The discussion continues as the energy flows, and the students are invited to describe what they feel.

"Warmth."

"A little tingling."

"Really relaxed. I could go to sleep."

When all the students have had the chance to feel what it is like to receive Reiki, we return to our chairs and continue talking about what it means to be able to practice this method of alternative healing.

34

Reiki is a Japanese word that is composed of two parts: *rei* means "Spirit-guided" or "soul-guided"; *ki* means "life-force." The most common translation of the name Reiki into English is "universal life-force energy." This translation acknowledges an important characteristic of the energy, which is experienced by everyone who works with it: universality. This energy is available to everyone, and is equally as powerful and effective in bringing healing to other species—and even to the earth itself—as it is in bringing healing to a person on the treatment table.

When you learn Reiki level I you are creating a new, broader foundation for your experience of life. Although when you leave the Reiki classroom, you may feel ready to try hands-on healing only on yourself or people close to you—your spouse or your best friend, perhaps—the effectiveness of the energy will soon encourage you to offer the help of your hands more often.

My first experience after learning Reiki level I illustrates how this can happen. I was in graduate school at the time I attended the class, and my mind was in the habit of critiquing and analyzing. When I completed the class I thought that my hands felt a little different, but I was skeptical that any real, lasting change had occurred. My intellectual mind could not grasp this possibility.

I practiced the hand positions rather haphazardly on myself for a few days. Then, wanting a break from my studies, I called my friend who lived on a Chester County farm, and asked if I could visit. She said that was fine but that I should be prepared to watch her paint while we talked, because she had a book-cover deadline to meet.

We chatted about all kinds of things—books and writing, boyfriends, career paths. She mentioned that she was quite upset about her horse, Holly, who was lame. My friend had spent all her savings—$750—on veterinary bills, and the vet could not tell her what was wrong.

There was my opportunity. "I just learned this thing—this method of hands-on healing—and if you are willing to hold the horse, I'll try it. I have no idea whether or not it will work."

"If it doesn't work, I won't have lost anything," she said. "I'll be glad to hold the horse."

We went out to the barn. As my friend held Holly's halter and stroked the horse's muzzle, she told me, "When you put your hands on the lame hoof, put them down firmly. Otherwise she'll think you are a fly and she'll kick."

That was enough warning for me. I knelt down slowly and planted both hands around Holly's lame hoof. Immediately I could feel my hands; I was so surprised! Even though I had left my Reiki level I class thinking that there might be something different about my hands, I had not expected the astounding range of sensation that I was now feeling: throbbing waves of energy across the hoof between my hands, tingles, whirls, heat. I "listened" to my hands attentively, fascinated.

After a while, my companion interrupted the silence. "Hey, look at that. Holly must like whatever you are doing. She's locked her back legs and gone to sleep."

Since I was unaware that horses sleep standing up, I had not noticed this shift in Holly's stance. I was glad that she found the Reiki relaxing. I was also relieved. There was now much less danger that I would be mistaken for a fly and get my hands crushed!

I stayed in the kneeling position with my hands on Holly's hoof for about forty-five minutes. It took that much time for the amount of energetic activity to diminish. I told my friend I did not know what the results would be, but that I would return, as I had been instructed to do by my teacher, at least a few more times over the next couple of weeks.

The next few times were much like the first. Holly was glad to see me, nickered at me in greeting, and stood quietly while I worked on the lame hoof.

Then, one day about a week later, my friend called. "Holly has thrown three abscesses from that hoof, and she's healing. The vet can't explain it. She's starting to walk okay again. I want to learn how to do Reiki."

The horse recovered beautifully, and over time her owner was able to ride her again for regular exercise and light work. My friend did learn Reiki, and is now also a Reiki master. And I recovered from my skepticism by considering how perfectly the universe had chosen my first client for me: a lame horse that could not be influenced by anything that I had to say about Reiki, whether skeptical or enthusiastic, but who could open to receive the benefit of the energy and use it to heal.

After that I was much more willing to offer Reiki to people. I no longer felt that I had to try to provide an explanation of something that was beyond my understanding. I became comfortable saying, "Look, I can't tell you how this works. It just works. Would you like to try it?"

My friend's cowriter, on a visit from San Francisco, let me work on his congested sinuses. After about twenty minutes he said, "I don't know what you are doing, but this is the first time I've been able to breathe through my nose in six months."

An eighty-four-year-old woman who is a family friend said that I could put my hands on her bad knee, which was swollen up with edema. After a while she said, "Don't take them away. They feel like a heating pad."

Taking advantage of opportunities to offer relief to familiar people and pets is a good way to begin to practice on others. People who are already in medical or allied medical professions will have many such opportunities immediately available to them; those who are not need to learn to recognize chances to be of service whenever they appear. Again, if your commitment is there, the universe will bring potential clients to your door—or will bring you to them.

THE PURPOSE OF REIKI

The meaning of the name Reiki that is closest to the Japanese, Spirit-guided (or soul-guided) life force, reveals something of the nature of the energy. A divine, infinite intelligence directs the healing process whenever you use Reiki. Your only effort is to place your attuned hands on yourself or someone else; when you do, the energy flows with an often startling intensity and power to accomplish acts of healing that are sometimes beyond the limits of the best medical school education, although perhaps not beyond the love and hope that live within the human heart. Sometimes Spirit-guided energy simply creates miracles.

Most of you will find, however, that Reiki is of value even when the results are not so miraculous. Being able to quickly stop the flow of blood from a nick made as you are shaving is mundane—and practical. Knowing that you can put your hands on your spouse's head for a few minutes and soothe away a headache is satisfying—and practical. Being able to do a couple of minutes of Reiki on yourself before an important business meeting is calming—and also practical.

It is in just such simple ways that most Reiki practitioners learn to integrate Reiki into their everyday lives. As they do, their lives begin to change, because their understanding has changed. Although being privileged to offer Reiki in a hospital setting can provide the chance to witness miracles, applying Reiki hands to a single cut flower in a vase and watching the flower perk up, glow with life, and then last much longer than other cut flowers also restores a sense of wonder.

Although no Reiki practitioner would take credit for a miraculous healing, Reiki practitioners can be glad for the opportunity to be of service and grateful for the privilege of working with this Spirit-guided power in whatever ways are open to them. Doing Reiki is soul-satisfying work—bringing comfort, relieving pain, cooperating with a force that always does good in the world.

The unexpected reward that this work brings is a greater sense of being guided in your own life to create healing for yourself and those around you. This might strike you in the form of a sudden inspiration to make a career change from corporate law to kindergarten teaching, but it is often more subtle than that: a day-by-day, moment-by-moment feeling of connection to spiritual guidance. With this sense of connection comes joy.

THE ATTUNEMENT PROCESS

During any traditionally taught Reiki level I class you receive four attunements or empowerments to channel healing. All four are exactly the same, and all four increase the flow of Reiki energy through your hands. However, because each attunement is transforming and has an impact on the body and the mind, an interval of time, usually at least two to two-and-one-half hours, is allowed to pass between attunements. This gives you the opportunity to assimilate the experience of the attunement, which can be gentle and calm or dramatic and emotionally intense.

From Hawayo Takata's account of her own First Degree Reiki class, Dr. Hayashi taught her and her classmates over four days.[1] Takata herself often taught Reiki I over three or four days. The Reiki masters Takata initiated, some of whom still travel internationally to teach Reiki, have often shortened the duration of the class, adapting their teaching plan to accommodate their students' five-day work week schedules. (My teacher, Rev. Beth Gray, consistently taught both Reiki I and Reiki II as full weekend classes; during a Reiki I class, the first attunement was given on Friday night, the second Saturday morning, the third that afternoon, and the fourth on Sunday afternoon.) Nowadays, few Reiki I classes are presented over such an interval of time.

Instead, traditional Reiki masters have had to make further accommodation to their students' schedules and to teaching venues. Many teach Reiki I as a one-day intensive and carefully time the intervals between the four attunements to allow students to integrate the energy they have received. Others, constrained by the requirement to standardize their class presentation to meet the needs of community college continuing education programs, teach Reiki I over four weeks, meeting for two or three hours one evening each week for a month. This allows students to receive one attunement at each class session and to practice Reiki between class sessions. This can be a real advantage, since students often find that besides having news of their first experiences with hands-on healing to share, they also have more questions about Reiki and how to "listen" to the energy in their hands.

Whatever the Reiki I class format and wherever the venue, traditional Western Reiki masters will repeat the attunement ritual that transforms the student into a channel for healing energy four times, as Hawayo Takata did, and as her teacher, Dr. Chujiro Hayashi did. The attunement ritual is sacred. It is at the heart of Reiki; the energy literally flows through the ritual to give the student healing and new life. The Reiki master is attuned to serve this purpose.

Traditionally taught Reiki masters hold the attunement ritual as not only sacred, but secret. For this reason, when I was first attuned by a Takata-trained Reiki master, I was led into a darkened room and asked to close my eyes and keep them shut during the attunement. This frightened me, and my fear colored my experience of the ritual.

However, I now understand the extreme measures taken to maintain the secrecy of the attunement ritual. Very simply, it should not be attempted by anyone who is not himself attuned as a Reiki master and trained as a teacher. Why not? For one thing, the amount of energy that can be transmitted through someone who is not a Reiki master is diminished. For another, someone who attempts to do an attunement without himself being attuned to the master level can find the experience causes considerable head, hand, arm, and shoulder pain, as energy attempts to travel through pathways that have not been sufficiently opened. This will lessen with application of Reiki hands to the affected areas. However, why risk uncertain, painful consequences to try such an experiment? This is an abuse of something sacred.

A certified Reiki master performs an attunement with a clear perception of its transforming nature and is able to offer the person attuned a strong foundation of spiritual understanding and emotional support. While holding the attunement ritual sacred, more and more traditional Reiki masters question keeping the attunement ritual completely secret and will talk with their students beforehand about what will occur.

My own first attunement might have been considerably different if what was about to occur had been described to me. My courage would not have faltered and my heart would have pounded less. Instead, without any explanation of what was about to go on, I attempted to follow instructions to the letter. With my eyes clamped shut, I endured the experience of the attunement in a frightened fury. Why, if this had nothing to do with religion, were my hands folded in the prayer position? This thought went around and around in my head. As a result, instead of seeing beautiful swirls of purple light like some of my fellow students, I "saw red." Only after returning to the main room and sitting for several minutes in quiet meditation with my fellow students did I acknowledge to myself that my hands might feel different.

When I look back at this experience, I feel sad. Although I know that my teacher was nobly honoring the vow of secrecy she had sworn to Takata, I would have been much more at ease if she had been able to offer some description of what was about to occur.

In order to spare my students from the distraction of a mind that is not at peace, in the classes I now teach I make a point of giving them a general description of the attunement ritual—what an observer to the class might see. I add that the mysterious and wonderful transformation that occurs during the attunement process—and much of the ritual itself—would not be visible to an observer.

Both the Reiki master and the students remove all jewelry, glasses, and shoes. Jewelry and glasses are removed because metal will attract the energy charge. It is the student who is to be attuned, rather than the student's jewelry. Shoes are removed so that energies can be grounded by contact with the earth.

The student is then asked to sit down in a chair, feet flat on the floor, hands joined, palms pressed together. The Reiki master may explain to the student that this hand position joins meridians in the fingertips and hands; it is also a position used throughout the world for prayer and meditation. In Japan, this hand position is called *gassho;* it has been used since Mikao Usui first taught Reiki in the 1920s to do meditation, to begin and end Reiki treatments, and to indicate readiness to receive an attunement. With the student's hands in this position, it is easier for the Reiki master to attune the heart and other areas on the front of the body.

The student is also told that her eyes may be opened or closed, but that she is likely to experience more of the subtlety and beauty of the attunement with eyes closed. This eases concentration and allows the mind's eye to see images and colors, much like the darkening of a movie theater's lights lets the movie seem bright and dramatic by contrast.

The Reiki master then stands in front of the student, feet flat on the floor, hands joined, and says a short prayer: When this prayer is completed, the Reiki master raises her hands, like a pair of antenna is raised to receive radio waves. And indeed, something much like this is actually occurring.

The Reiki master walks counterclockwise behind the student, lowers her hands to the student's head in a gesture of blessing, and asks for spiritual permission to proceed. When this is received, the Reiki master puts one hand up and, with the other, makes a series of symbols over the crown of the head. This opens the energy center in the head to receive the high, healing Reiki energy.

Then the Reiki master circles around to stand in front of the student again. The Reiki master takes the student's joined hands in one of her own; with the other hand she draws symbols into the heart area, the throat, and the forehead.

Finally, the Reiki master separates the student's joined hands and slaps them, one at a time. She places the right hand, after it is attuned, on the student's left shoulder, and the left hand, after it is attuned, on the student's right shoulder, so that the student can begin to feel the flow of Reiki energy from the hands into the body.

When this step is completed, the Reiki master continues her circle to stand again behind the student. Here, she says a prayer of thanksgiving and rejoicing for the student's empowerment with the Reiki energy. This ends the attunement ritual.

When I complete an attunement, I walk around to face my students and tell those who have their eyes shut that they can open their eyes whenever they want. Then I ask if anyone would like their eyeglasses returned to them. Next, I offer a glass of water to assist the student in coming back to ordinary awareness; it provides a cool, clearing sensation through the center of the body that is grounding.

I then ask the students what they experienced.

*"I felt a sense of pressure when you stood right in front of me, and then when you
walked away, I began to see different colors. Then, when you stood in front of
me again, I felt my hands get hot."*

*"I don't know if I felt anything different. My fingertips feel a little tingly. That's
all, though."*

"I heard a gong sound and I saw this really beautiful purple light."

*"There was this flash of white light. Then there were all the colors of the rainbow.
It was really spectacular."*

*"I felt heat in the back of my head, on one side. It still feels warm. I can feel a
pulsing in my fingertips."*

"I don't feel any different. Is that okay?"

It is okay. The first attunement can provide an extremely powerful opening for a student who is ready for such an opening. This is rare, though. Most
people have some mild sensation of energy flowing through their hands or in
their heads, but some feel no difference at all. This is fine. The energy becomes
more apparent with each subsequent attunement.

REIKI HANDS

If you have had the opportunity to experience a Reiki treatment, you know that
it is quite relaxing and soothing. This may be your reason for wanting to learn
Reiki—to provide this gentle experience for clients, or for family and friends.

Your perception of the experience of receiving a Reiki treatment may also
be much more precise and detailed. You may have felt comforting warmth
under the practitioner's hands or extending outward in all directions from the
practitioner's hands; you may have been aware of tingling or waves or a soft
flow of the current of healing energy. You may also have felt intense heat or a
sense of mild pressure or movement, even though the practitioner assured you
he was not doing massage and his hands were still. This may have been accompanied by the simple recognition that your breathing had become easier, your
pulse steadier and stronger, your digestion faster.

As a newly attuned Reiki practitioner, you will now experience such sensations as the energy flows through your attuned hands. The sensations you experience will be natural, and many of them will feel familiar to you already. You know what a change in the temperature of your hands feels like; you know what tingling feels like from rubbing your hands together briskly to keep them warm on a cold day; you recognize the sensation of "pins and needles," similar to what happens when you stay in one position so long your hand becomes numb and "falls asleep." All of these sensations of the flow of energy in your hands are familiar and easy to describe.

With each attunement you receive, however, your hands are going to become stronger, steadier channels for the flow of healing energy. You will register this flow of energy in these familiar ways, and in some new ways that are natural extensions of the ways you already know. For example, you may be used to thinking of your hands as presenting a small range of surface temperatures: most of the time they are warm, but when you are in a room with the thermostat turned down in the winter, your hands become quite cold. Now, with each attunement, the range of surface temperatures is going to become greater. Your hands will usually be noticeably warmer or cooler when you are providing a treatment. At times your hands may feel so hot that even the air above them seems hot, as if they are surrounded by a cloud of radiant heat. On other occasions the heat may seem so concentrated under your palm that you feel as if you were holding your hands near a match flame. When you experience such sensations, you may also find that your palms are actually perspiring.

Such temperature differences will help you to recognize the sensations you are experiencing as an expression of the flow of healing energy. At times the sensation of warmth or heat is not limited to the hands, but seems to travel all the way to the shoulders and the torso. This is indicative of a strong need on the part of the person receiving the energy.

Perhaps surprisingly, the sensation of cold or coolness can also indicate the flow of healing energy. At times this is pleasant and refreshing to the practitioner; at other times it is simply something to accept in the spirit of service. The sensations experienced are not of the practitioner's choice; they are expressions of the healing energy flowing through the practitioner's hands to meet the needs of the client. When the energy is needed in a different way, it modulates itself in answer to that need, and the practitioner notices a subtle or a marked shift.

Another familiar sensation that you may experience is tingling or "pins and needles." When this is how the healing energy expresses itself, the sensation will be sustained for some time—as long as the area of the client's body under your hands is calling for the energy—but it will not be uncomfortable to you. You will often be able to isolate the locus of the tingling precisely. You may say to the client, "I feel a tingling under the knuckle of my right index finger" or "The base of my palm up to my wrist seems prickly." This is an accurate description of your perception of the energy. In time you will learn that such specific sensations are informative about the client's condition.

Some sensations will seem new to the practitioner. For example, after a short time most practitioners experience the sensation of energy being pulled or drawn down into the client's body. Another common sensation is that of a vortex or whirlpool of energy, often under a fingertip or a finger joint. Sometimes practitioners also feel a wave of energy moving gently back and forth between their hands.

Again, although most people have not felt these sensations in their hands with ordinary touch, they have felt similar sensations while sitting in a tub with their fingers gently waving in the water or with their toes in the whirlpool flow over the drain. These are common ways we perceive the effects of energy (in the bathtub, the energy of motion in a liquid medium).

As you learn Reiki, such sensations become familiar, comfortable, and meaningful. You learn to listen to your hands, which will speak now with a greater expressiveness than you have ever experienced before. The cognitive change may be compared to learning the alphabet for the first time. Although many people learn how to use enough letters to write their own names before they go to kindergarten or school, suddenly having all twenty-six letters in their repertoire and seeing them in combinations that are increasingly familiar allows them to begin to read. As a Reiki practitioner, you will have an increased sensitivity to energy and a heightened perception of the sensations accompanying energy flow. In time, you will learn not only to listen to your hands, but to "read the body" under your hands like the blind read Braille—as a language that makes a whole world of understanding possible in new and meaningful ways.

The first step is to register the energy flow through your hands as you do the hand positions for Reiki on yourself. After receiving only one of the four attunements that open your hands to channel the energy, you may not feel much in terms of sensations of energy flow. However, with each additional attunement, and with practice, your awareness will greatly increase.

When you first put your hands on yourself or someone else after your first attunement, the energy will begin to flow and your hands will be "on." Since you are not used to the energy yet, you may not even notice. After a few minutes, however, the energy will have had a chance to flow into you and relieve some of your points of stress; after this, the energy will begin to flow *through* you. Because your hands have been opened through the attunement, you may begin to notice some mild sensations—a gentle increase in warmth, perhaps, or a little tingling in your little finger, or a pulsing under a knuckle. Be patient with whatever you are feeling, and keep listening, concentrating on the sensations. Over a few minutes' time they will build to a higher level of energy activity than you have experienced before—beyond your old, familiar, range of sensation. Then this level of energy activity will plateau for whatever period of time the body needs to "refuel" with energy for healing. When the level begins to drop off, you can move your hands to another position.

Whether you work on a client or yourself, whether you are doing a full treatment or "Band-Aiding" a hurt, this is the basic pattern of energy flow you will listen for in your hands: a single, complete cycle that begins with contact, increases to noticeable activity, builds to a plateau, and then drops off when a therapeutic amount of energy has been received.

After some practice you will learn that the degree of activity in your hands corresponds to the degree of health or injury or disease, or to the acute or chronic nature of a condition. An old but severe injury will call forth a strong draw of energy, particularly if the injury did not heal completely or well. An acute condition may create an intense but brief and complex level of activity; a chronic condition will also create an intense level of activity, but for a considerably longer period of time. Although your hands will tell you that an area is the site of severe, acute, or chronic pain, they will not tell you when the injury occurred, when the disease was contracted, or when a condition became systemic. The energy is not limited by our concepts of linear chronological time; for example, if an old knee injury from ten years ago needs healing even more than a day-to-day stress-related condition, such as a headache, then the level of energy activity in the hands will be stronger over the site of the old knee injury than over the head.

As you become comfortable with this new sensitivity to the flow of energy through your hands, you will discover yourself making statements and asking questions that surprise you. "I feel a sharp line of energy activity that crosses my knuckles. It is different from what I am feeling in the rest of my hand. Could this have been the site of an injury?" you may ask. The client will often confirm your impression by saying something like, "Yes, I fractured that bone playing baseball when I was a kid," or "I had surgery in that area several years ago. It's amazing that you feel that."

It *is* amazing, and also absolutely normal, for you to experience this degree of sensitivity to the flow of energy. The Reiki attunement literally expands your conscious awareness: your sensitivity to energy is increased; your external senses, primarily tactile and kinesthetic, are sharpened; and your internal connection to higher consciousness, particularly through the intuition, is strengthened.

For this reason, many Reiki practitioners find doing a treatment on themselves or someone else moves issues of personality out of the way; cooperating with the channeling of healing energy is consciously consenting to a stronger spiritual connection, even if only for a moment. This experience feels meditative, even though the focus of the meditation is not the breath but the hands, and the purpose of the meditation is not spiritual enlightenment but practical healing.

WORKING ON YOURSELF AND OTHERS

Although you may be interested in Reiki primarily because you are a caregiver and wish to bring greater healing to those you care for, once you learn Reiki, remember to work on yourself every day. Why? There are many good reasons: You will be better prepared to cope with both crises and ordinary stress. Your sense of wellness will have a tonic effect on everyone around you. When you care for others who have a medical condition, an injury, or an illness, your solid foundation of health will enable you to help them without feeling overwhelmed. You will enjoy feeling well yourself. And the most practical reason? Reiki energy flows more quickly through a practitioner's hands to those he wishes to treat when he is healthy.

While many of us have been brought up to believe that it is more blessed to give than to receive, the practice of Reiki shows that giving and receiving healing energy are both blessings, meant to be enjoyed in balance. Reiki works by flowing through a channel, but in order to flow through, it must first fill up. When you require more healing because you are under stress or are not feeling well, the energy will go first to reduce your stress and symptoms—not relieving them altogether, but diminishing their importance to your conscious mind. Then the energy will begin to flow through your hands to your client. In other words, your stress and discomfort delay both the sensation of the flow of healing energy through your hands and the start of the actual sending of healing energy to the person who has come seeking treatment.

Stress will also slow the sending of the healing energy even when you are simply treating yourself. If you have a bad day at work and decide to do a Reiki treatment on yourself as soon as you get home, you may discover that your hands seem slower to "turn on" than they did in the morning when you treated yourself. This delay may only be momentary, if you are consistent in doing daily self-treatment, or the delay may be for five or ten or even twenty minutes, if you have fallen out of the habit of doing Reiki each day or the stress you are enduring is extreme. Be patient when this happens. Once you have received the fourth and final attunement of your Reiki level I class, you have Reiki hands for the rest of your life. The energy begins to flow as soon as you place your hands in position on yourself, or on someone else, with the thought of providing treatment; however, it will always address your need for healing to some degree before you feel its flow through your hands.

As an example, one evening when I was visiting a friend who was showing his work in an art festival the next day, I had the opportunity to work on someone who was suffering from an impacted wisdom tooth. I had been up since five o'clock in the morning, and had been busy all day helping my friend set up his booth and make other preparations. I drank a lot of coffee through the day to keep going. By the time I was asked to treat this man's toothache, it was one o'clock in the morning and I could hardly keep my eyes open. Rather than attempting to do a full treatment, I placed my hands on the man's face, over the aching area. I waited. Nothing happened. Ten minutes went by; still I could not feel the flow of the healing energy in my hands. Then we were interrupted, so I broke off the contact and apologized that I had been unable to ease the man's discomfort. A few minutes later my friend, who also knew Reiki, came into the room and offered to continue the treatment. Immediately his hands turned on, and he was able to provide this man with relief from pain. My friend is a confirmed night owl and is often just going to bed when I, a morning person, am getting up. The next day, after a decent night's sleep, my hands turned on as quickly as they usually do—within seconds of making physical contact. In the wee hours of the morning, however, when I was exhausted, they were not quick to do so. I might have waited another five or ten minutes before the Reiki energy circulating in me was sufficient to ease my sense of stress and course through my hands, but because we were interrupted, this did not occur. This delay in the sending of healing energy can occur whenever there is some extreme stress on the practitioner, even when the practitioner is very much in practice.

Normally the flow of Reiki energy begins with physical contact. There is a saying in the Reiki community: "Hands on, Reiki on." The sense of flow through the hands is immediate and easy to perceive for a practitioner who treats herself and others daily. However, the flow begins with physical contact even for a practitioner who does not practice daily or who is in poor health or under extreme stress. For these practitioners, the flow will be directed first to those areas of their own bodies that need healing. This may or may not be accompanied by perceptible sensations of energy flowing to those areas. When the healing energy begins to flow through the hands, however, the practitioner will soon become aware of this activity.

Daily self-treatment can help you get healthy and stay healthy, maintain a positive mental attitude, and step forward on your own spiritual path. In listening to your hands each day as you treat yourself and others to Reiki, you are listening to Spirit-guided life-force energy. You witness something sacred, vital, dynamic, and healing. This has the power to touch the heart like an answer to a prayer.

Reiki is so practical, however, that it is also easy to place in a real-world perspective. It is a tool, a skill that many people learn to help them cope with seasonal colds and runny noses and children's banged knees at soccer games. Reiki need not be at the center of a person's life to be of value; even given only a few minutes a day out of a hectic schedule, it remains gently transforming.

USING STANDARD POSITIONS
FOR TREATMENT

In most traditional Reiki classes, twelve positions are taught to provide a complete Reiki treatment; they may begin on the head or on the front of the torso, but they support healing to all the major organs and systems of the body. In addition, there are also many extra positions that you may use to treat yourself or a client who requests them.

The twelve standard positions that I was taught by my teacher begin on the front of the torso, continue at the head, and conclude with the back. These hand positions provide a comprehensive treatment of the major organs and systems of the body. They are simple and easy to do, whether you are treating yourself or a client. The positions evolved from those Takata learned from her teacher, Dr. Hayashi, who paired practitioners together to treat patients in his Reiki clinic in Tokyo in the 1920s and 1930s. These positions may easily be performed comfortably and effectively by a single practitioner.

As I was taught, I teach my students to begin on the front of the torso. However, there are times when it is clearly appropriate and fitting to begin on the head. For example, if the primary complaint is a sinus condition and this is causing stress, sending Reiki first to the blocked sinuses (covered by the first hand position on the head) may bring relief more quickly and effectively than sending Reiki to the adrenal glands (covered by the first hand position on the torso), which release adrenaline to help us cope with stress.

I believe that it is a good habit for every Reiki practitioner to begin hands-on treatment with the first hand position taught by his teacher and to break from this tradition only when his own need or the need of the client urgently recommends this course to the conscious mind. This is definitely not a matter of letting the placement of your hands be guided by intuition; it is a matter of attending to a strongly presenting symptom in the most practical and healing way. For example, in treating a sufferer of childhood epilepsy, prone to frequent seizures, it makes sense to begin treatment on the feet to balance and steady the erratic energetic misfirings occurring within the brain; in treating a client with congestive heart failure, it makes sense to treat the heart first to stimulate circulation into the rest of the torso, the head, and the extremities. Yet a

Reiki treatment done entirely in standard hand positions will bring benefits.

The twelve positions described in the following chapter allow a complete and effective treatment to be delivered to the major organs of the body in a time-efficient way, whether the positions are begun on the front of the torso or on the head. Arms, legs, hands, and feet also receive some Reiki energy during and after such a treatment, because the Reiki energy goes to wherever it is needed in the body.

Although there has been no scientific determination as to the exact process through which this distribution of healing energy occurs, it seems safe to assume that Reiki uses the circulatory and nerve pathways to disperse itself throughout the body; it seems equally clear to practiced Reiki hands that the energy is not limited to these pathways. The sensation of the energy traveling from the torso to the toes, for example, can be quite noticeable. When you are working on yourself, you may feel this disbursement as a moving line or band of warmth or tingling radiating out from under your hands to another area of your body; if you are working on a client and the client becomes aware of a similar movement of energy, she may rouse herself from a relaxed state to comment on the effect. "Every time you move your hands, I feel a surge of energy down my right leg," she might say. "This is the leg that has been bothering me so much since the accident I was in last spring."

Since Reiki goes where it is needed, and a complete twelve-position Reiki treatment allows this to occur, most practitioners do not spend time doing extra positions on themselves unless they have a special reason to do so. The same principle applies when a practitioner works on a client: The twelve standard positions are sufficient for a complete treatment, but if both practitioner and client have time and the desire to do so, extra positions on the upper chest area, throat, and extremities may be done for added healing benefits.

Reiki offers you the opportunity to bring healing to yourself and others on all levels of being—physical, emotional, mental or psychological, and spiritual. The satisfaction that comes from seeing yourself and others enjoying better health, realizing creative talents, and pursuing dreams cannot be measured. Ultimately, you may use Reiki to find your happiness, for happiness and health go hand in hand.

4

WORKING ON YOURSELF WITH REIKI

A complete daily self-treatment includes sending Reiki energy from each of the twelve standard positions, beginning with the four positions included in Basic I, on the front torso; continuing with the four positions included in Basic II, on the head; and ending with the four positions included in Basic III, on the back. Although these standard positions (and some extra positions) are described here with some degree of anatomical detail, it is not necessary to know anatomy to treat yourself or anyone else with Reiki. By simply laying your attuned hands on the body and listening to the flow of energy, you can know clearly what areas need to be treated and how long you should hold each position.

THE BASIC HAND POSITIONS

The best way to learn the twelve standard hand positions is to see them demonstrated in a quick walk-through in class, to register the placement and the movements. Once you are sure of the positions, you can try a walk-through yourself, not concerning yourself with sensations of energy, but simply practicing how to place your hands. Once you have the positions down, you can do them more slowly, taking the time in each position to listen to your hands and feel the flow of Reiki's healing energy come on, increase to a steady level of activity, and then gradually or suddenly decrease, signaling you to move to the next position. This allows the body to receive the amount of energy it naturally calls for to provide an energetic foundation for healing to occur, to stabilize, and to begin to build. This is accomplished by listening to your hands, rather than by looking at a clock or attending to the voice of your intuition, to decide that your hands have been in any one position long enough.

Like many practitioners, you may decide to set your alarm clock to go off at an earlier time in order to treat yourself first thing in the morning; or you might enjoy using Reiki on yourself just before you go to sleep. The Reiki energy will go through pajamas or nightgown and sheets, so there is no need to make any special preparations. Just wake up in bed or get ready for bed as you normally do, put your Reiki hands on, and relax. Do not make it a goal to "get through" all the positions. It is better to treat even one position with deep Reiki healing than to race through a treatment without paying attention to the energy's gentle, soothing flow. Allow yourself to be present to your experience, to appreciate what is occurring, and to be grateful.

Basic I, Position 1 (Figure 4.1)

The first position used on the torso of the body covers most of the lower rib cage. To mark the top line of this position, find the end of the sternum or breastbone, just above the soft flesh over the diaphragm. You should be able to feel a small area of thicker bone under your fingertips (see figure 4.2 on page 54). On some people this bone, called the xiphoid process, may be knobby, and so is found quite easily; on others it is fairly flat and difficult to find. If you search with your fingertips and cannot easily locate the xiphoid process, simply go to the bottom of the breastbone and use this as your starting line.

To treat yourself in Basic I, position 1, lay the right hand flat, palm down, thumb against palm and fingers together, over the lower right side of your rib cage, just under the breast if you are female or the pectoral muscles if you are male. At the same time, lay your left hand flat, palm down, thumb against palm and fingers together, over the lower left side of the rib cage, so that the

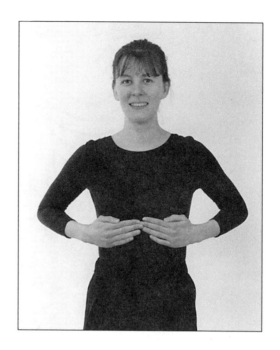

Figure 4.1

fingertips of the left hand meet, but do not overlap, those of the right hand along the vertical centerline of the body. When you place your hands correctly on yourself in this position, you will find that they comfortably and lightly wrap around the front of the lower part of your chest.

Your Reiki touch here will benefit the bones of the lower rib cage, the diaphragm, the lungs, the liver, the stomach, the pancreas (behind the stomach), and the spleen. Behind these organs the adrenal glands and the kidneys will receive the energy's healing effects. The blood supplied to these organs from the heart through the abdominal aorta and other major arteries will be washed in the energy's healing flow, before it circulates throughout the body and back to the heart. The nerve pathways to these organs from the spinal cord will be sparked with the impulse to accelerate all natural processes that are healing: for example, digestion will speed up and blood sugar levels will stabilize more quickly.

Because Basic I, position 1 covers some of the organs most sensitive to stress, many Reiki channels favor it for creating a feeling of relaxation and will discover ways to send themselves this soothing flow in stressful situations. For example, during a business meeting a Reiki channel may sit with her arms crossed over her chest—not to signal "I'm closed off" to her business

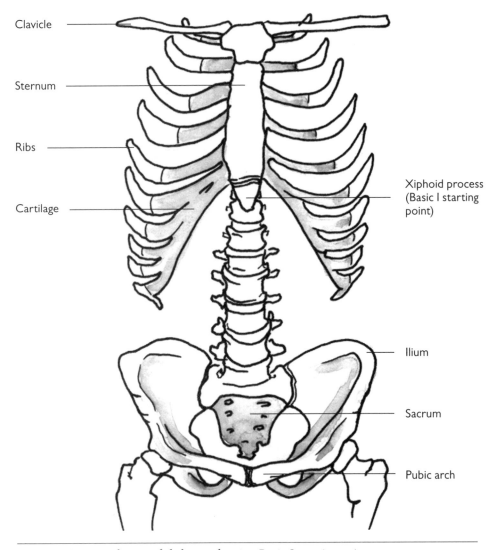

Clavicle

Sternum

Ribs

Cartilage

Xiphoid process
(Basic I starting
point)

Ilium

Sacrum

Pubic arch

Figure 4.2. Frontal view of skeleton, showing Basic I starting point

colleagues, but simply to feel the relaxing sensations of the energy flow relieving her tension.

Reiki channels who do a treatment on themselves before they go to sleep
at night often relax so deeply with their hands in Basic I, position 1 that they
drift off to sleep without ever moving their hands to the second position. This
is, perhaps, not startling; what is startling, however, is waking several hours
later to discover that you have slept on your back, elbows out like wings, with
your hands in the first position, and you have slept well and feel refreshed and

clear. This is an interesting contrast to the findings of sleep researchers that the average adult turns some twenty times a night during sleep.

Basic I, Position 2 (Figure 4.3)

On a person of average height and weight, the second position used on the front of the torso spans the area from the bottom of the rib cage to just above the waist. Of course, not everyone is of average height and weight. In the first position a tall, long-waisted, or heavy person may find his hands resting high above the waist; a short or short-waisted person may find her hands are already close to her navel. Wherever your hands are in Basic I, position 1, Reiki will allow you to move through the standard positions and adapt them for your unique physical body with ease. If you are tall, for example, you may simply do more hand positions to cover the torso than your much shorter spouse. If you are short, you may do fewer hand positions to cover the torso than the standard method for self-treatment suggests.

To move from Basic I, position 1 to the next position, note where your little fingers are placed, then drop your hands down a single hand-span. Your fingers should be relaxed but touching one another, your thumbs against the knuckles of your index fingers, your palms flat. You are now in Basic I, position 2.

Under your hands (from the bottom of the rib cage to just above the waist), the organs of the body that will be receiving direct benefit include the lower

Figure 4.3

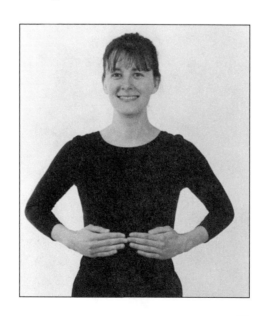

part of the stomach and the liver—both large organs. Behind them, the common bile duct and the cystic duct join the pancreas with the gall bladder, which is sheltered under the liver. The intestines begin with the duodenum descending from the stomach to the jejunum and the small intestine, and the transverse colon—part of the large intestine—wrapping over the duodenum, as if protecting it. In the center of the body, in front of the spinal cord, major arteries and veins circulate the blood flow to and from these organs and from the kidneys. The ureters begin their descent from the kidneys to the urinary bladder, draining the body of fluid waste products.

Like first position, Basic I, position 2 is another important focus for stress relief. As our language reveals, the emotions we experience in response to stressful events are often played out here in our bodies. Many people talk about "swallowing their anger," "getting butterflies in the stomach," or simply complain of "a nervous stomach." Reiki soothes, calms, relaxes—and as the physical body responds, so does the emotional body.

Basic I, Position 3 (Figure 4.4)
This position is the "belly laugh" position. The area usually spanned is from just above the waistline to just below the waistline, with fingertips meeting over the belly button or navel.

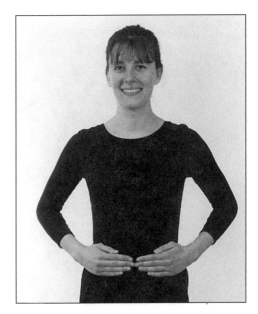

Figure 4.4

To move from Basic I, position 2, to Basic I, position 3 is easy: again, notice the position of your hands, especially your little fingers, and then drop down a hand span. When you settle into the new position, keep your hands relaxed and your touch light, but do hold your fingers and thumbs close together so that you will be able to deliver the Reiki energy in a concentrated manner. Under your hands, beneath the soft skin of your belly, the mass of the small intestines and parts of the ascending colon on the right and the descending colon on the left will receive the direct benefit of Reiki energy. The kidneys, which float rhythmically up and down about ten inches, may float downward with exhalation into this area; the ureters, which descend from the kidneys to the urinary bladder, will be bathed in the energy's healing flow. The inferior mesenteric artery carries blood into this area from the heart, and the inferior vena cava circulates the blood back. Lesser arteries and veins and many nerve pathways support this area of the body as well. As you leave your hands in this position to give yourself Reiki, you may have sensations of the energy radiating out, following these pathways to other parts of the body.

Basic I, Position 4 (Figure 4.5)

The final position in the Basic I group covers the lower part of the abdomen, just within the pelvic cradle to the tip of the pubic bone. This position is easy

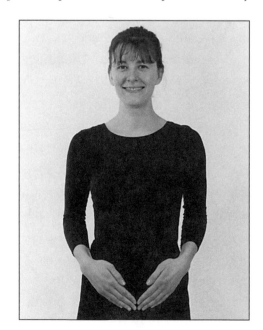

Figure 4.5

to move into without lifting your hands up; simply slide them down until they come to rest naturally in a V just inside your hip bones. At the bottom of the V your fingertips will still touch, but your hands will not span your abdomen in a straight line. They will slant downward, following the body's natural contours. With your hands in this position, the Reiki energy will flow directly through your skin and abdominal muscles to your intestinal tract. Under your right hand will be the ascending colon (part of your large intestine) and your appendix; under your left hand will be the descending colon. If you are female, your thumbs, index, and middle fingers of both hands will be covering your ureters and urinary bladder, as well as your ovaries, fallopian tubes, part of the uterus, cervix, and vagina. If you are male, your thumbs, index, and middle fingers will be covering your ureters and urinary bladder, as well as the prostate gland, the seminal vesicles, and the vas deferens. Beneath the urinary tract and reproductive organs, the sigmoid colon, the last segment of the large intestine, which descends to the rectum, will also receive Reiki energy.

Like many Reiki channels, you may find this position quite comforting, whether the flow in your hands in this position seems even, like a blanket, or is more subtly varied. A Reiki channel who has either had a baby or undergone a hysterectomy may feel differences in the energy flowing through her thumbs and index and middle fingertips, which lie directly over the reproductive organs, and the ring and last fingertips, which lie directly over the urinary bladder. The differences may be quite surprising at first. Eventually the flow will even out and shift to a lower level of activity, a signal from your body that it has enough energy to do healing and that you may move to the next position—either Basic II, position 1 (on the head), or an extra position on the front of your body. (Possible extra positions are described in chapter 5.) Allow the energetic sensations in your hands, more than logic or intuition, to guide you in making this decision. If Basic I, position 2 had a strong energy draw and you know that you have recently been exposed to the flu, you may want to move your hands to the extra position over the sternum (described in detail on page 72), which covers the thymus, the endocrine gland that produces infection-fighting T cells (see figure 4.6). Or if you noticed that Basic I, position 4 drew heavily and you are premen-

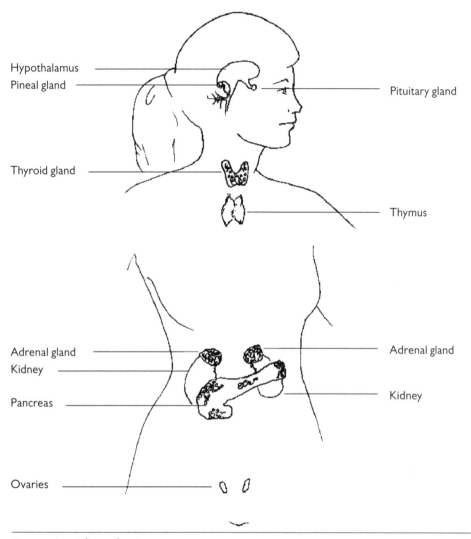

Hypothalamus
Pineal gland
Pituitary gland
Thyroid gland
Thymus
Adrenal gland
Kidney
Pancreas
Adrenal gland
Kidney
Ovaries

Figure 4.6. *The endocrine system*

strual, you may want to consider doing extra positions over the center of the abdomen, directly over the uterus.

Even without doing extra positions, through consistent daily self-treatment using only the twelve standard positions, you will do wonders to maintain your sense of well-being through all the body's natural cycles. Day after day the energy will disperse itself to wherever it is needed, whether or not you can perceive it doing so. This is a tremendously powerful way to guard your own health.

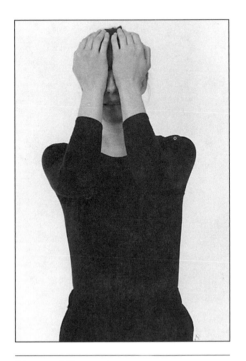

Figure 4.7

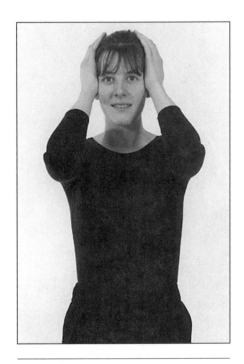

Figure 4.8

Basic II, Position 1 (Figure 4.7)

Basic II, position 1 covers the forehead, eyes, part of the nose, and the cheekbones. The position is as simple as playing peekaboo—raise your hands up, fingers together, thumbs pressed against palms, and place them over your eyes palms down, so that they meet in the middle of your forehead, the little finger of the right hand meeting the little finger of the left hand and the palms separating naturally over the nose. The base of the palms should be level with the bottom of your nose.

This position covers skin tissue, muscle, forehead (frontal) bone, eye sockets and eyes, nasal bone, septum, sinuses, and the maxilla, the bone that serves to anchor the upper teeth. It also covers the front of the cerebrum, which includes the frontal lobes of the left and right cerebral hemispheres—the part of the brain that governs the abilities of language-making and comprehension, problem-solving, and various aspects of personality.

Doing Reiki on yourself in this position is a natural and effective way to relieve headache pain. It can also provide comfort and ease symptoms of a head cold, an eye or sinus infection, a bout of hay fever or allergies, or any infection that affects the upper respiratory system. It is also a good "wake-up call" for tired eyes and mind, and can help stimulate mental alertness.

Basic II, Position 2 (Figure 4.8)

To move from Basic II, position 1 to Basic II, position 2, use your thumbs as position markers.

Swing your hands out (as if showing yourself during peekaboo) and then touch little fingers to thumbs. Lift up the thumbs and allow your little fingers to mark the front edge of position 2. Rest your hands against your temples and cheekbones, palms flat, fingers straight and together, thumbs against palms. Feel the flow of Reiki energy through the area on the sides of the head.

Under your hands—under the skin of your temples, your cheekbones, and your scalp—the frontal, temporal, and parietal bones of the skull meet on each side of the head, and the frontal, temporal, and parietal lobes of each of the brain's two hemispheres come together. Here, the brain makes sense of motor and sensory information. Nerve and blood pathways to the eyes, nose, ears, and mouth traverse these areas. In particular, the trigeminal cranial nerve, responsible for facial sensations and muscle movements, branches out over the surface of the scalp, around the eye socket to the eye and nasal cavities, and along the jawline.

Deeper within the skull, but still accessible to the energy, the optic nerves, messengers of visual sensory impressions to the brain, travel from the back of the retina of each eye to a crossing point called the optic chiasma (just in front of the pituitary gland) into the cerebrum. Deeper still, running parallel along each side of the cleft that joins the two hemispheres, the olfactory nerves travel to and from the olfactory bulbs, relaying information about smells.

Here, under the optic chiasma, behind the sinuses, the pituitary gland (master gland of the endocrine system), the thalamus (a regulator of emotions), and the hypothalamus (a mediator of messages from the hemispheres regarding stress) nestle together, controlling the release of hormones for healthy growth, metabolism, response to stress, and reproduction.

Doing Reiki on yourself in this position helps bring biochemical imbalances back into healthy balance. Daily treatments help maintain this balance to keep the body well. Again, sending Reiki in this position is helpful for acute eyestrain, headaches, and sinus congestion from colds or other infections or allergies, as well as for more serious conditions involving brain function, hormonal function, or mental and emotional disorders.

Basic II, Position 3 (Figure 4.9)

Moving from Basic II, position 2 to Basic II, position 3 is accomplished in the same way as from position 1 to position 2. Using your thumbs as position

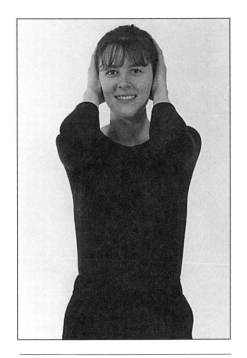

Figure 4.9

markers, swing your hands out and then touch little fingers to thumbs. Lift up the thumbs and allow your little fingers to mark the front edge of position 3. Relax your hands against the sides of your head, so that your palms cover your ears. The fingers of each of your hands should be touching, and your thumbs should be against your palms. You are now in Basic II, position 3.

The most important sensory organs under your hands in this position are, of course, your ears, delicate spirals of flesh and cartilage that funnel sound through the ear canals to the eardrums, which vibrate against the mechanisms of the middle and inner ear to transmit sound impulses along nerve pathways to the brain (see figure 4.10). The fluid-filled labyrinthine spirals of the inner ear also contain tiny free-floating particles called otoliths, which, like the needle in

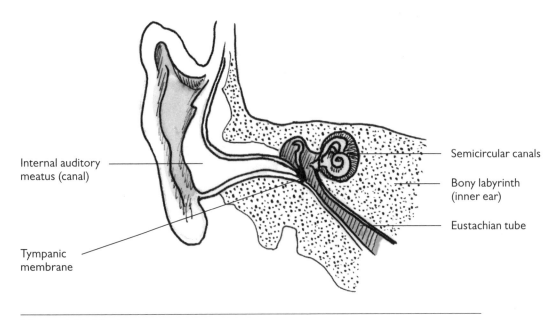

Figure 4.10. *The inner ear*

a compass, help us find our body's "true north" by constantly registering our position in space. This information also follows nerve pathways to the brain.

The back of the nose and mouth passageways—the sphenoidal air sinus, the eustachian tube (a tiny canal that equalizes air pressure on both sides of the eardrum and that connects the ear to the throat), and the soft palate— are also under your hands in this position, as are nerves that register smell, taste, and tactile sensations on the skin of the face. The temporal and parietal lobes of the brain arch together over the midbrain cavity and its essential array of endocrine system regulators: thalamus, hypothalamus, pituitary, and pineal glands.

Reiki hands applied in this position can help to heal ear infections, including the viral infections that cause labyrinthitis. Nasal congestion can be loosened, sore throats soothed, cold-deadened sense of taste restored, and a wide variety of allergies allayed. More serious conditions affecting the brain or the regulating mechanisms deep within the brain may also receive needed healing through Reiki hands applied here.

Basic II, Position 4 (Figures 4.11 and 4.12)

Basic II, position 4, covers the back of the head; although you may treat this area effectively with your hands held vertically (figure 4.11), as you have for the other positions in Basic II, it is much easier on the wrists to use your hands horizontally, so that you cradle the back of the head (figure 4.12). If you choose to hold your hands vertically, move into this position as you have before, "walking" your hands around the head and then settling into position. Depending upon the size of your head and your hands, and the thickness of your hair, your hands may or may not be touching along the vertical centerline of the back of your head. If not, simply slide them together so that they do meet, or add an extra position.

If you prefer to cradle the back of your head, this is fine. As you move from Basic II, position 3, over your ears, into this position, stack your hands, one on top of the other, so that the back of your head is completely covered. It does not matter which hand sits on top. What does matter is that you can send healing energy to yourself in this position without causing undue stress in your neck, shoulders, or wrists.

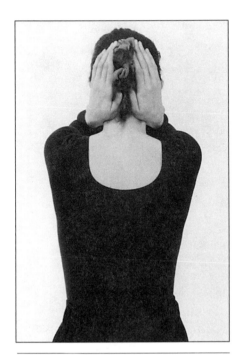

Figure 4.11

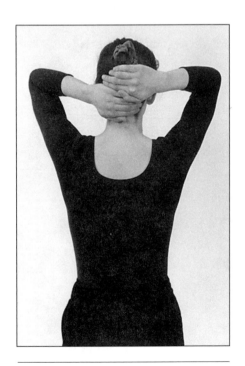

Figure 4.12

With your hands in either of these positions, you will be directing Reiki energy into the back of the cerebrum and into the cerebellum, the reptilian brain that controls many of the survival mechanisms we developed on the way to becoming *Homo sapiens*. Many of the autonomic nervous system functions absolutely essential to life are controlled from here.

With a little practice and some opportunity to work on yourself or others who are fighting infections, you will also recognize that many immune system mechanisms appear to be triggered by this area of the brain. Because of this, Reiki to this position seems to do a great deal of good for anyone who is fighting an infection or who has a suppressed or compromised immune system. Paired with a Reiki hand applied across the forehead, a hand here, over the back of the head at the base of the skull, will quickly ease most headaches.

If the alternate position seems comfortable to you and you recognize it as one you have already used during a languorous stretch, after a couple of hours at the computer or in the library carrels, you will not be surprised to learn that it can be used to boost physical and mental alertness.

Basic III, Position 1 (Figure 4.13)
Basic III covers the back, and the first position used is exactly opposite the first position of Basic I, on the torso, over the lower rib cage. To reach the bottom line of this position, bend your elbows and reach behind you as high as you can before letting your hands come to rest a few inches

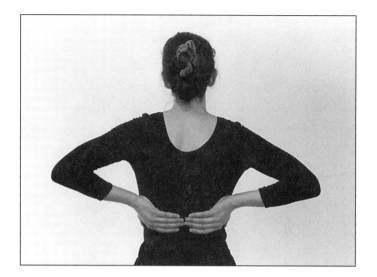

Figure 4.13

below your shoulder blades. Ideally you will be able to keep the fingers of each hand together to form a wide band to deliver the energy, but you will need to use your thumbs against your sides to brace your hands high.

Although you may not find this a comfortable position, do your best to lay your hands as flat as you can against your back. You will be covering the bottom of the trapezius muscle where it tapers over the lower thoracic spine, and the long, wide bands of the latissimus dorsi muscle that stretch over the ribs and up to the underarm. Nerve pathways at this level branch out from the spine, relaying messages to and from the diaphragm, kidneys, pancreas, spleen, stomach, and liver. Surface- and deeper-level veins and arteries branch out to the organs in this area from the vena cava and the aorta, which run parallel to the spine, circulating blood to and from the heart. The adrenal glands, perched atop the kidneys on each side of the spine, are accessible here. Most Reiki channels find considerable relief from stress by sending healing energy to these "fight-or-flight" hormone producers, which are called upon quite often in our fast-changing, high-tech, high-tension times.

Basic III, Position 2 (Figure 4.14)

To move from Basic III, position 1, with hands palms down and thumbs braced against your sides, to Basic III, position 2, slide your hands down a single hand-span. This position is considerably more comfortable for most people

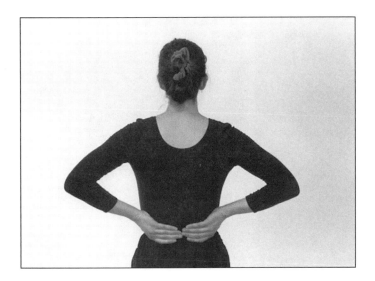

Figure 4.14

than the first, and as a result, once your hands are attuned to Reiki you may find yourself adopting this easy pose whenever you have the opportunity.

Under your hands (from the bottom of the rib cage to just above the waist), the energy will penetrate first through muscle, bones, nerves, veins, and arteries, to some of the major organs of the urinary and gastrointestinal tracts—the kidneys and ureters, pancreas, gall bladder, liver, stomach, and parts of the intestines.

As with all the standard positions on the back, they echo in placement the same position on the front of the torso. If you have been thorough in your Reiki treatment of yourself to this point and listened to the energy in your hands surge on, maintain a steady level of activity, and then shift to a diminished level of activity, you may discover that your back needs very little Reiki, because it has already received it while you did the hand positions on the front.

Basic III, Position 3 (Figure 4.15)

This position spans the area from just above the waistline to just below the waistline, with fingertips meeting along the centerline of the body, over the lower back. Basic III, position 3 is as easy to do as Basic III, position 2. From the second position, slide both of your hands down the back a single hand-span, allowing your thumbs to wrap around your waist.

In Basic III, position 3, your hands will direct the energy through the skin to the muscular fascia over the latissimus dorsi and the sacrospinalis—long, large muscles over the lower back, spine, and sacrum that support flexing and twisting movements. If you do not actively exercise, however, you may recognize them as the muscles that carry the greatest tension for you—the ones people reach for when they say, "Oh, my aching back!" Under these muscles, where the vertebrae of the spine widen out, nerves, veins, and arteries support the urinary, gastrointestinal, and reproductive organs.

Anyone with a tendency toward kidney infections or kidney stones will be able to feel the energy level increase as the kidneys float downward into this area. Pregnant women and women who are premenstrual or menstruating will find that the application of Reiki hands in this position can bring great relief from muscle aches and cramps. Leave your hands here through several cycles of energy flow to bring even more lasting relief.

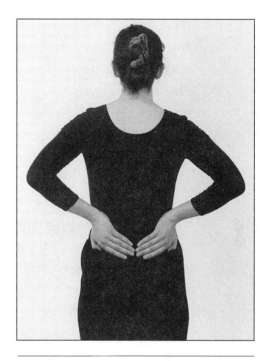

Figure 4.15

Basic III, Position 4 (Figure 4.16)

Like the fourth position in Basic I, the fourth position in Basic III is very easy to do. From the third position, where your hands rest at waist level against your lower back, slide your hands downward in a V. Pull in your thumbs so they are against your palms. Your fingertips will meet at the bottom of the V over your sacrum, the large triangular bone at the bottom of the spine. This bone, the "keystone" of the pelvis, sits between the hip bones (the ilia) and allows for pelvic motion.

With your hands in this position, energy

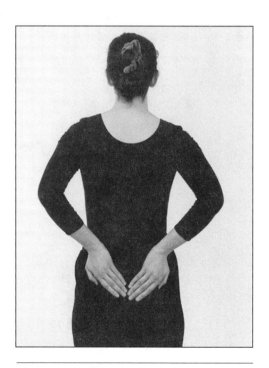

Figure 4.16

flows through skin, muscle, and the hollow channels of the sacrum to the sciatic, sacral, gluteal, and pudendal nerves. These support lower limb, urinary tract, gastrointestinal tract, and reproductive system functions. Just in front of the sacrum, the vena cava and the aorta, which run parallel to the spine to this point, divide into the external and internal iliac veins and arteries. These supply the blood flow to the abdomen, the hips, and the legs and feet. The intestines, the reproductive organs, and the bladder nestle forward of these veins within the pelvic cradle.

Working on yourself in this position provides a pleasant antidote to sitting for too long. The energy can penetrate more deeply, of course, to aid in relief of intestinal cramps, diarrhea, constipation, or bloating. Relief can also be obtained from the lower back pain that comes with premenstrual tension, menstruation, or pregnancy. This is also frequently the site of old injuries, some of them dating back to childhood falls. Reiki hands here can soothe the body's memory of such traumas, like a lullaby can put a cranky baby to sleep.

As you begin to work with Reiki, your new commitment to healing is likely to serve as a catalyst to quicken any change you want to make toward a healthier lifestyle. For example, if you have wanted for some time to quit smoking or lose weight and have been unable to do so, you may now discover that you possess the willpower you need.

If you have already made changes to create a healthier lifestyle and are in good health, working on yourself will strengthen your sense of vitality and brighten your mood. A healthy body will not call for much Reiki energy, so you will discover that you can do a treatment on yourself in as little as ten to twenty minutes each day and maintain a high level of wellness.

If you are in generally good health with some minor complaints, you will find that initially you need to self-treat for slightly longer than your healthier friends or spouse. However, as you start to treat yourself hands-on with Reiki consistently each day, aches and pains that have been with you for a long time will begin to diminish in intensity and duration. Eventually they will disappear, and you will simply feel well. When you reach this point, you, too, will be spending only a short time in self-treatment each day, for wellness is easier to maintain than minor imbalances are to correct.

If you have a chronic or progressively debilitating condition, your daily Reiki treatment on yourself will require some time—perhaps as long as forty-five minutes or an hour once or twice each day. The results of your investment of time will be gratifying, though. Initially, you are likely to experience the alleviation of your most severe symptoms and a reduction in pain for short periods of time. Then, with consistent daily self-treatment, milder symptoms will start to come under control, and you will live pain-free for longer and longer intervals. Eventually you may go into complete remission or the diagnosis of "incurable" may be reversed, as evidenced by blood levels of antibodies and antigens and other medical tests. For this to occur, however, you must be as committed to your daily Reiki self-treatment time as you are to following whatever regimen your medical doctor has prescribed. (Reiki's gentle method of sending Spirit-guided life-force energy to the physical body—and all levels of being—will complement a prescribed regimen and may bring about healing where Western physicians no longer expect healing to occur, but only hope to ease the discomfort of symptoms. This is because Reiki treats the cause of illness and debilitating conditions, not merely the effects.)

Good health is a blessing, and being able to maintain good health with the help of your own Reiki hands is a blessing and an empowerment. Self-treatment has immediate positive effects, as well as subtle aftereffects that will play out in your life through the course of the day, and sometimes even for a few days following. In addition to feeling physically better, you will find yourself smiling more often and laughing more easily. People around you may behave with more kindness and consideration, and circumstances that concerned you may seem to fall into place. This is striking, especially at first, and may seem somewhat mysterious.

Why is the universe suddenly offering you so much cooperation? Giving yourself a Reiki treatment changes your energy in a positive way. You become much more likely to attract positive people and experiences to yourself when you (and your whole aura) are charged with the light, loving quality of Reiki energy. This is in complete harmony with Reiki's purpose of healing. Through daily self-treatment with hands-on Reiki, you send healing to yourself. Your healing brings healing all around you and, for those who come to you asking for healing, your healing makes theirs proceed more quickly and easily.

5

OPTIONAL POSITIONS FOR SELF-TREATMENT

Although a complete Reiki self-treatment, practiced daily in the privacy of your home, will do wonders for your health and sense of well-being, from time to time you may want to do some extra positions to focus healing on a particular site of muscle strain or tear, bone break, infection, incision, or other injury outside the areas directly covered by Basic I, II, and III. While no particular hand placements are required to do extra positions, some are suggested here for the comfort of the practitioner and because they have been shown to be appropriate for certain common conditions. (For less common conditions or diseases that manifest symptoms at several sites in the body, do a complete treatment and site-specific extra positions as your understanding guides you.) All of the extra positions can be done fully clothed, and a few can be done discreetly in public. For example, lots of Reiki practitioners drive with one hand on the wheel and another on the thymus. While I do not recommend this as a safe driving practice, I commend the sensibility that realizes the value of applying Reiki whenever the opportunity arises—that is, whenever at least one hand is free.

As part of daily self-treatment, you may do one or more extra positions after completing all the standard positions, or you may integrate the positions into the treatment by adding extras for the front of the body to Basic I, for the head to Basic II, and for the back to Basic III. Whether you do these extras before or after the Basic I, II, or III group will depend upon physical symptoms and comfort level.

BASIC I OPTIONAL POSITIONS

Heart (Figure 5.1)

The heart may be treated by using the same gesture that Americans use to pledge allegiance: a hand placed gently over the left side of the chest, palm down, fingers together, thumb pressed against the palm. For troubling indigestion or heartburn symptoms, one hand placed above another may be even more soothing. If the symptom feels quite concentrated, you may stack your hands, one on top of the other, to increase the flow of energy to the area and relieve the pain.

Because the heart circulates blood throughout the body, any blood-borne infection or condition, including autoimmune system disorders such as allergies, may be particularly helped by focused treatment on the heart. Electrical shock victims may also be restored more quickly to proper fluid-electrolyte balance by direct application of Reiki to this area.

Figure 5.1

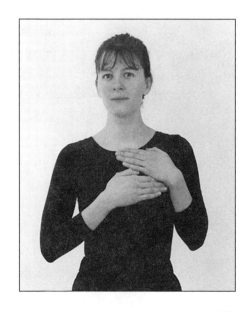

71

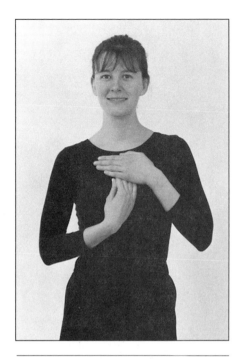

Figure 5.2

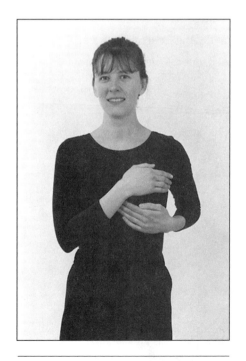

Figure 5.3

Thymus T (Figure 5.2)

At the top of the sternum, secure behind a thick wall of bone and covering part of the heart, is the thymus, a much misunderstood organ whose important role in fighting infection is now becoming recognized. Because the thymus is large in children and shrinks to a fraction of its original size in adults, it was once thought of as vestigial and was readily removed. The thymus cranks out T cells, a type of white blood cell considered to be so essential to a strong immune system that T-cell count is monitored regularly in AIDs patients. Even those who fight an infection of a much milder nature, such as a cold or flu, can benefit from application of Reiki hands here. By placing one hand horizontally just below the collarbone and the other hand vertically over the sternum, you can treat the thymus.

Breasts (Figure 5.3)

To maintain breast health treat both breasts individually, using enough hand positions to make a full circle of healing energy. (Your hands can tell you if there is any change in your breasts' condition. If you suspect a cyst or tumor, continue to Reiki your breasts often, and see your doctor as quickly as you can for an examination and mammogram.)

Recovery from surgical incisions in this area can be greatly speeded up with the application of Reiki hands. By crossing your arms and tucking your hands in your armpits, you can also treat the many lymph nodes in this area for improved infection-fighting and wound drainage.

Since people come to Reiki at every stage of life, and in all states of wellness and illness, you may discover that Reiki plays an essential part in your recovery from a lumpectomy or mastectomy. Allow yourself to become more educated about physical, mental, emotional, or environmental factors in your lifestyle that may have triggered the onset of your disease. Use what you learn to make any necessary and positive lifestyle changes that you can manage to stabilize your healthy recovery and enhance your self-esteem. Love yourself unconditionally, let the flow of healing energy through your Reiki hands bring you hope, and move forward with joy in life.

Upper Respiratory Tract (Figure 5.4)

Anyone suffering from a cold, bronchitis, or other upper respiratory tract infection knows how congested and uncomfortable this area can become. Asthma sufferers, whose bronchial passages tighten and sometimes close during an attack, must deal with much more severe and dangerous symptoms. Laying the hands lightly over the upper chest area, either in an upward pointing V or one above the other across the upper chest, eases the sense of congestion of a cold or bronchitis. The same position, used daily by an asthma sufferer, may gradually reduce the frequency and the severity of attacks. (The way to check the reversal of symptoms, however, is not to throw away your bronchodilator, but to see a medical doctor on a regular basis and have lung

Figure 5.4

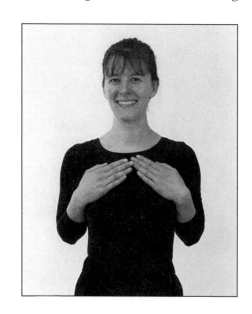

Reiki Level I

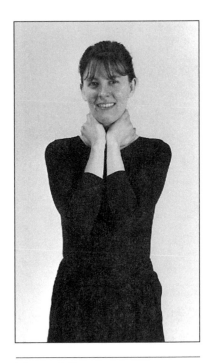

Figure 5.5

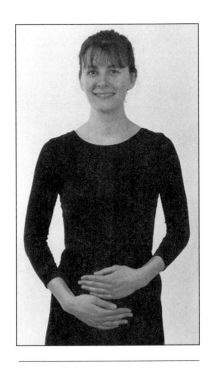

Figure 5.6

capacity carefully monitored until the doctor releases you from her care.)

Throat (Figure 5.5)

The throat may be treated from Basic I or from Basic II. One easy way to treat this area is to sit with your elbows on a table and your hands arched around the sides of your neck. Your throat, thyroid, and parathyroid glands will receive Reiki energy from the base of your palms, and salivary and lymph glands will feel the flow from the upper part of your palms and your fingers. This is such a soothing position to perform that many Reiki channels find ways to do it for long periods of time—say, while at the movies—by draping one hand comfortably over this area in what looks like a habitual gesture.

Abdomen (Figure 5.6)

After doing Basic I, position 4—the V just inside the pelvic cradle—it is easy to move the hands parallel, one above the other, over the center area of the V. This directly targets the reproductive organs, and so can ease menstrual pain and the pain of labor contractions. If you are pregnant, it is also a lovely way to direct healing energy to your baby.

"Hinges" (Figure 5.8)

Where the torso joins the leg, the femoral arteries supply blood to the lower extremities from the heart, which is pumped back on its return journey through the femoral veins. For this reason, anyone who has reduced circulation to the legs or feet will want to send Reiki energy to the hip folds or "hinges."

Many lymph nodes are situated along this same

curve (see figure 5.7). Anyone fighting an infection, particularly one that has affected any of the organs within the abdominal cavity, will want to apply Reiki hands here. This will aid in both the production of new antibodies to maintain

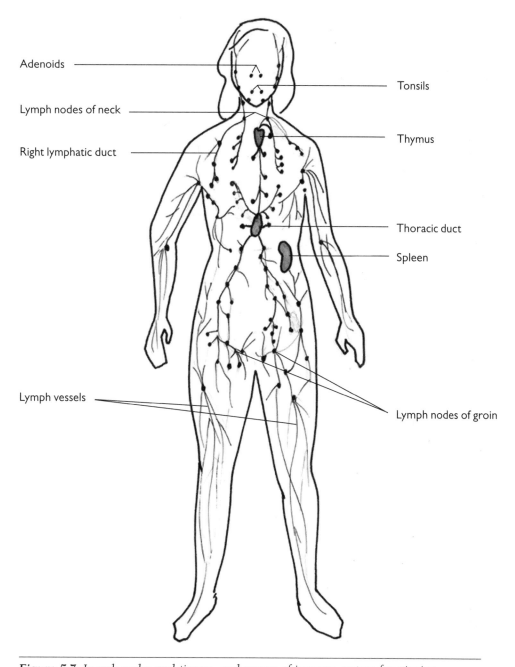

Figure 5.7. *Lymph nodes and tissues, and organs of immune-system functioning*

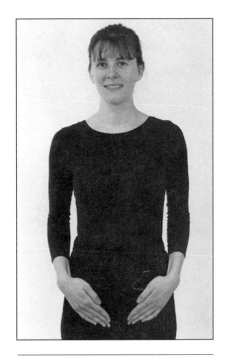

Figure 5.8

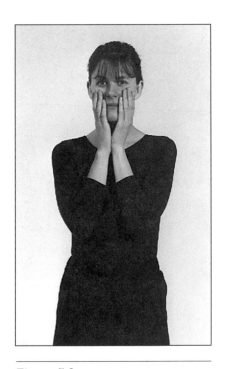

Figure 5.9

the fight, and in the destruction and disposal of the invading organism or foreign substance.

To do this position, simply slide your hands from the V of Basic I, position 4 a few inches downward on both sides, forming a wider V over the place where the legs meet the torso. As always, listen to your hands to determine the length of time to spend in this position. When the energy shifts to a lower level of activity, move on.

BASIC II OPTIONAL POSITIONS

Lower Front Face (Figure 5.9)

While most people will find extra positions on the head unnecessary, anyone who has occasional allergies or sinus infections will enjoy the soothing quality of hands-on attention applied to the sinus cavities in the lower part of the face. For those people who "can always tell when a storm is coming" because the changes in barometric pressure affect their sinuses and teeth, this position can also provide much needed relief.

To do this position, simply place your hands, palms down, under your eyes, leaving a space for your nose. The knuckles at the top of your palms will lay over your lower jaw, or mandible. Your thumbs will naturally curve along the lower jaw. This is an easy position to do sitting down, with your elbows on a table or desk. You may also find this position comfortable to do while sitting on a couch, with a pillow upright in your lap to provide support under your arms.

Jawbone and Teeth (Figure 5.10)

Allergy and sinus condition sufferers can tell you that the dull ache they experience is localized to particular areas of the head and neck. This is largely because the principal nerve pathways to the face divide into branches that run over the crown of the head, over and under the eye, and down from the top of the ear along the jawline. For this reason, these people can obtain some symptom relief by applying Reiki hands consistently over the jawbone (mandible) and back teeth (molars).

The easiest way to do this extra position is to sit with your elbows on the table and support your head with your hands. Let your chin rest comfortably and naturally in the curved hollow of your hands. Then allow the healing energy a few moments to penetrate and soothe. If you stay with the flow of the energy through the first downward fluctuation, the healing energy will go even deeper.

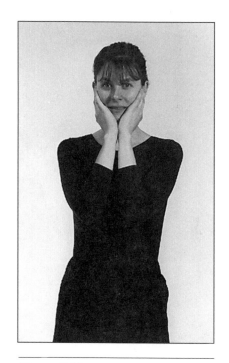

Figure 5.10

Neck Area Under Ears (Figure 5.11)

Massage therapists will tell you that pain in the face is often accompanied by trigger-point pain in the sternocleidomastoid muscles, the long muscles that begin just behind each ear and broaden into a wider band, near the collarbone. These muscles overlie the carotid arteries and the two jugular veins, the major channels of blood circulation to and from the brain. They also shelter a number of lymph nodes that produce antibodies and drain infections' residues from the tissue.

Reiki hands applied over this area are comforting indeed, and can be placed in position while seated at a table, elbows resting on the table surface,

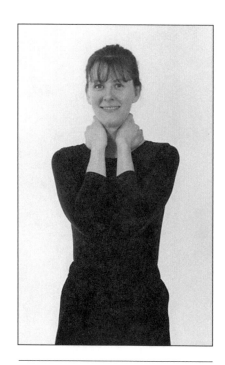

Figure 5.11

77

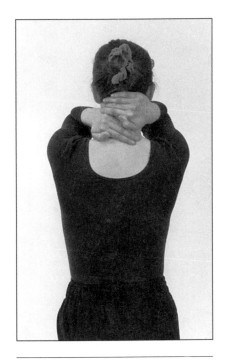

Figure 5.12

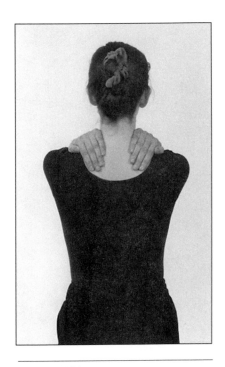

Figure 5.13

or while doing a standing or seated shoulder-stretch. Healing energy here can ease trigger-point pain and relax related muscle tension, drain lymph nodes, and clear congestion from head colds, allergies, and ear infections. This can relieve the painful sense of pressure and "pop" the ears open so that there is a return to normal hearing.

Back of the Neck (Figure 5.12)

Reiki hands applied parallel, one above the other, on the back of the neck are helpful for easing muscle tension and tension headaches. Because they penetrate to the nerves that exit from the cervical vertebrae, however, they can do much more. They can speed relief to herpes simplex sufferers who have lesions on or inside the mouth or nose, or who suffer from herpetic neuralgia; and they can sometimes prevent the onset of lesions if applied at the first sign of an outbreak—a slight itching or mildly painful swelling sensation at the site. Herpes sufferers may be tempted to substitute Reiki for prescribed medication, such as acyclovir ointment or tablets. Instead, please do as your doctor prescribes, and allow Reiki to be adjunct therapy, at least until such time as your immune system has recovered sufficiently that your doctor recommends another course of treatment.

BASIC III OPTIONAL POSITIONS

Shoulders (Figure 5.13)

The top of the shoulders are tension traps for many people in today's society—a rough day at the office usually translates into stiff, contracted trapezius muscles. Short of heading to the gym or the pool or the tennis court for a warm-up and a workout, or to an appointment with a massage therapist, you can do a lot to relieve stiffness and ache here by applying Reiki hands where it hurts.

You can work on your shoulders by letting your hands come to rest on them, right across those tensed trapezius muscles. You can also treat your shoulders one at a time, simply bending your arm at the elbow, lifting your arm high, and letting your hand drop down comfortably onto the shoulder on the same side. A few minutes' break from your work to Reiki yourself in this position can make the rest of the day much more pleasant.

Sciatic Nerves (Figure 5.14)

People who are troubled by sciatic nerve pain are well aware of the route that these thick bundles of nerves take in exiting the bottom of the spinal column. They will reach for the lower back and point to two little indentations on each side of the back of the pelvis. "This is where the pain begins," they will explain. "And it continues out along the hip and then down the side of the leg."

The sciatic nerve is not one nerve, but several nerves that branch off of the lower spine and sacrum. Each nerve follows an L-shaped pathway as it exits from the spinal cord and crosses the back of the pelvis, then joins the composite nerve

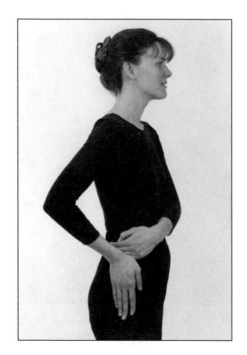

Figure 5.14

bundle (called the lumbosacral plexus) to travel down each leg. The sciatic nerve bundle branches at many points, providing sensory information to and from the groin, the thighs, the knees, the shins and calves, the ankles, and the feet. It is for this reason that people often experience sciatic pain not only in the lower back and across the back of the hip, but at sites much lower down the leg.

Treating your own sciatica is mostly a matter of being aware of the route the sciatic nerves take, and remembering that Reiki applied at the cause is even more effective than Reiki applied to the site of referred pain. For this reason, it is normally sufficient to treat this problem with extra hand positions diagonally in a V across the lower back (over the indentation in the pelvis) and vertically from the indentation in the pelvis down the sides of the legs.

OPTIONAL POSITIONS FOR THE EXTREMITIES

Arms, Elbows, Wrists, Hands (Figures 5.15, 5.16, 5.17)

If you have a site of an acute muscle strain, injury, or infection in your arms, wrists, or hands, applying Reiki consistently will speed healing. Since you will

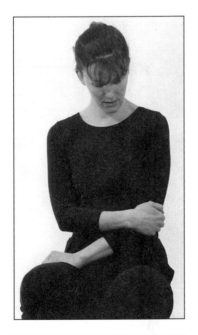

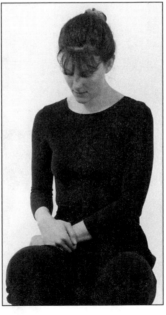

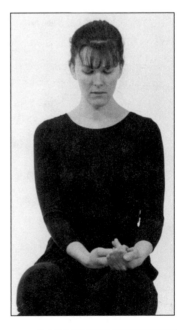

Figure 5.15   *Figure 5.16*   *Figure 5.17*

work one-handed on yourself, be as comfortable as you can in using the available Reiki hand. Circle joints gradually, listening for shifts in the energy. Cover strained, swollen, or torn muscles or ligaments until the flow diminishes in activity.

Remember that pain in shoulders, elbows, and hands can be referred pain from repetitive stress injuries or carpal tunnel syndrome. Although some relief may be obtained from applying Reiki where it hurts, work on the affected tendons and ligaments in the wrist is usually necessary to bring about the rapid recovery practitioners come to expect with Reiki.

A cut or burn on the finger of one hand can be treated with the other hand. If the Reiki energy feels too hot over a burn, you can lift your hand and work an inch or two above the burn, still with good healing results.

Legs, Knees, Ankles, Feet
(Figures 5.18, 5.19, 5.20, 5.21)

You may, from time to time, want to treat a strained or torn muscle, tendon, or ligament, or a cut across a muscle with Reiki and will find that it is easy to do so simply by applying your hands over the affected area. If, however, you are interested in healing knees or ankles that have sustained athletic injuries, whether old or recent, you will discover that there is benefit in sending Reiki to the affected joint from all sides. You can usually treat the knee comfortably simply by sitting with your knee slightly bent. A fully bent knee with the foot supported will give you comfortable access to the ankle. If you are in a cast, sit and gently bend down from the waist. Apply your hands over the injury site and listen. Despite the cast, the Reiki energy will turn on and flow through to the area where it is needed.

Feet are often neglected until problems develop. Something you can do to pamper your feet is to Reiki them while you are in a warm bath. Your muscles will be relaxed, and you will probably be able to bend comfortably from the waist and reach the soles of your feet with ease. The Reiki energy flowing into your feet is very relaxing when added to the warmth of bath water.

The other way to work on your feet is one at a time: sit with one leg knee to chest so that your heel is braced on the edge of your chair and your foot is roughly arm's length away. Or sit with one leg bent at the knee, lifted up, and

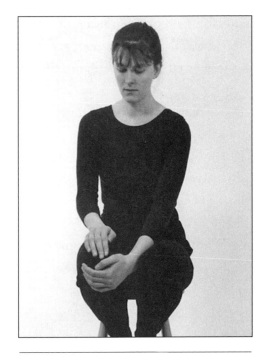

Figure 5.18

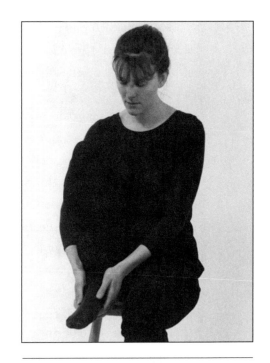

Figure 5.19

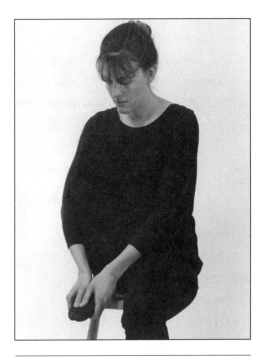

Figure 5.20

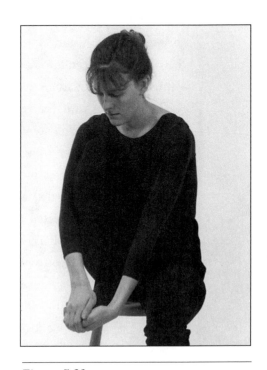

Figure 5.21

crossed over the opposite knee, so that your foot can comfortably rest, again at arm's length. Do lots of hand positions to provide thorough healing to this hard-working part of your body, which, according to reflexology, has energetic connections to all your major organs. There is something wonderful about feeling like you are "walking on air."

PRACTICING THE HAND POSITIONS

Depending upon how the level I course is taught, whether over one, two, three, or four days, students may have the chance to practice the pattern of hand positions for self-treatment in class and then directly after class, as "homework." The assignment is simple: work on yourself, using the standard positions and any extra positions that seem appropriate, as you go to sleep. Although you may have had only one attunement at this point, it is still quite possible to feel the flow of the Reiki energy in each position and to benefit from its healing effects.

This is what you may notice as you listen to your hands for the first time. As you place your hands in Basic I, position 1, you may feel nothing at first or you may feel an immediate mild warmth or faint tingling. Whatever you feel is fine. Keep listening. In a few minutes you may notice a gentle flow of healing energy. This means that your hands have turned on. Simply leave your hands in this position and notice the sensations that you feel. Remember that you may feel mild warmth, a comfortable coolness, or intense heat or cold; you may also feel tingling, prickles, whirls, or waves; or a sense of pressure, pull, or draw. These sensations all indicate the flow of energy and are all normal for anyone with Reiki-attuned hands.

After several minutes you are likely to feel the flow of energy change, noticeably diminishing *or* significantly increasing in intensity and level of activity. A shift in either direction is a signal that the area under your hands has absorbed enough energy to begin the work of accelerated healing, so that you may move your hands to the next position with confidence that you have provided sufficiently thorough treatment.

If you allow your hands to stay in position after such a noticeable shift, you will soon feel the Reiki energy begin another cycle. When this happens, the energy is penetrating to an even deeper level of tissues and organs, supporting the body's healing even more.

However, *usually* the change you will feel after several minutes of treating yourself (or a client) with Reiki is a decrease in intensity or level of activity. Because this is the case, in the pages that follow, you will be reminded to shift your hands to another position when you feel an ebbing of the flow, a quieting of the sensations in your hands, or a decrease in activity. Consider even a slightly noticeable reduction in the flow a sufficient signal for you to move your hands to the next position.

In Basic I, position 2, allow your hands to stay in this position until you feel the complete cycle of the energy flow turning on, actively sending healing, and then quieting. Go through as many positions as you can, listening for your hands to turn on, send healing, and then turn off (or at least turn down). You may find that going through the positions this way, as you lay in bed before sleep, is so relaxing that you drift off into deep, restful sleep and dreams. That is fine. A good night's rest will prepare you well for the next class session.

6

THE ORIGIN OF REIKI HEALING

As the students arrive for the next session of the Reiki I class, they search for familiar faces and smile shyly at new friends. They chat easily with one another as they find their chairs. Finally, the Reiki master welcomes them with a bright smile and invites them to share their experiences a bit more formally. She calls on each student in turn to ask about their success with their "homework" assignment: to do Reiki on themselves in bed at night, before they fall asleep. She asks one student, "Did you get through all the hand positions?"

"Well, no. I think I fell asleep as soon as I hit the pillow. I did put my hands in the Basic I, first position, and I woke up in the middle of the night to find that I hadn't moved. But I don't remember feeling the energy."

The next student has a different report to make:

"I cleaned my kitchen until two o'clock in the morning. And then I tried to use Reiki on my cat George, who was already asleep on my bed. He didn't wake

up, but he did sort of stretch out like he was really enjoying it, and he purred. Then I got into bed and I did all the positions of Basic I. When I got to my head, I rolled over on my side and just went to sleep. I think I did feel my hands, though. Tingling."

"I gave my wife a massage. I could feel my hands on her back felt really hot. She said it was great. She fell asleep, and then I was awake. I watched the late news and did the positions on myself as I watched TV. Was that okay to do?"

The Reiki master nods and smiles, and invites another student to speak.

"I just did the positions and I didn't feel much. But I did try to listen to my hands, to feel them go on and then send healing and then turn off. I think I could feel that pretty clearly in the third position, but I'm not sure about the others. I had great dreams, though. I woke up this morning and I tried to do the positions again, and everything seemed much clearer. Maybe I was just tired last night."

"My hands were hot. I was really amazed. I have diabetes, and I've been working on myself with traditional and alternative medicine for years to try to get better. I'm in the habit of using a healing meditation CD as I go to sleep. So I put that on the CD player the way that I usually do, and then I got in bed and put my hands in the first position. I never imagined that my hands could feel that way! Something was really happening. So I just kept them there. I kept listening for the energy flow to decrease, but I don't think it ever did. It just kept increasing. So I fell asleep like that. And today I feel great."

"I wish something like that had happened to me. I really feel unsure of myself. I know I felt energy in my hands during and after the attunement, but when I put them on myself in the hand positions last night, I couldn't feel much of anything. I couldn't tell if what I was feeling was warmth from my hands or warmth from my own body. I hope I can feel my hands more clearly today."

Whatever experiences the students report, the Reiki master can assure them that every sensation of the energy that they feel is fine. The opening to channel Reiki energy through the process of the four attunements is gentle and gradual. Although some students are very open and sensitive to the strength of the Reiki energy flow after only one attunement, this is fairly rare. Most people need all four attunements to feel confident that they can "listen to their hands" and recognize the energy's healing cycle.

RECONNECTING TO UNIVERSAL LIFE-FORCE ENERGY

When the Reiki master attunes students the second time, she repeats the steps and symbols for a level I attunement. Student responses vary considerably.

> *"That was intense. I saw this flash of light when you slapped my hands. Now they are still tingling, as if you just slapped them a second ago."*
>
> *"I could feel this pulsing sensation between my palms the whole time."*
>
> *"I felt a kind of lightness in my head, and then I saw this incredible turquoise color like you see in advertisements for Jamaica. And then I felt this bouncing sensation in my hands."*
>
> *"I saw my dog. His name is Ralph, and he's just a puppy. He really seemed to like my hands last night. I think I want to give him some healing."*
>
> *"I saw this place where I go to do meditation. It's in a lovely green woods, and there's a waterfall there, and a fountain."*
>
> *"My palms are sweating now."*

Just as with the first attunement, whatever sensations the students report are fine. Sometimes there is little noticeable difference from the first, and sometimes there is quite a lot. What is important to understand is that the energy is being delivered to you exactly where you are. Whether you have been open for years to ideas about alternative healing and spirituality, or closed until coming to the Reiki class, the energy will meet you, uplift you, and help you move along your own path at a pace that is healing for you.

As you listen to the Reiki master tell the story of Reiki, remember: "Don't waste your hands." Put your hands on your thighs or over your belly. Cross your arms and tuck your hands against your sides. Sit with your hands folded. Begin to get in the habit now of using the Reiki energy flowing through your hands for your own healing.

THE EARLY HISTORY OF THE REIKI METHOD

You may wonder how Reiki, which is so different from traditional Western medicine, came to be taught in this country. In fact, Reiki is taught not only here and in Japan but all around the world, in many different languages, to people of all races, all nations, all religions and creeds. To understand how the teaching of Reiki came to be so widespread, it will help to learn something of its history.

The "Usui method of natural healing" was first practiced and taught in the early 1920s in Japan, by Mikao Usui (August 15, 1865–March 9, 1926). While not much about Mikao Usui's early life is known, a glance at his portrait suggests he was a person of refined intelligence, sensitivity, and gentleness. His expression seems at once stern and tender—appropriate for a man whose life demonstrated both spiritual discipline and compassion for all humankind. Most accounts of his life agree on the single, most significant event: Mikao Usui sought enlightenment through a twenty-one-day meditation, fast, and prayer vigil on Mount Kurama, a sacred mountain just north of Kyoto. His spiritual awakening, at dawn of the twenty-first day, was accompanied by an extraordinary transformation: Mikao Usui could perform healing through the touch of his hands. He used this ability first to heal himself and then to heal others, eventually treating thousands of people throughout Japan. Many of those he treated were eager to learn this gentle hands-on healing method themselves. He gladly taught them Reiki.

Among those who regarded Mikao Usui as a spiritual teacher and healer and who helped to develop Usui's Reiki method of natural healing into a teachable system was Dr. Chujiro Hayashi (September 15, 1879–May 10, 1940), a physician and retired naval officer. Usui requested that Dr. Hayashi establish a Reiki clinic in another location from the center where Usui treated people with Reiki and taught. Hayashi honored his teacher's request and opened a Reiki clinic in Yotsuya (now Shinjuku ward), Tokyo.[1]

Dr. Hayashi maintained this clinic even after Mikao Usui's death in 1926 and treated many patients who often went on to become Reiki practitioners themselves. Soon, because of Reiki's effectiveness, the clinic had a wonderful reputation. News of its success with difficult cases reached people all over Japan, including even some doctors and surgeons at other well-known medical centers.

In fact, in 1935, when the widowed and sickly Hawayo Takata (December 24,

1900–December 12, 1980) traveled to Japan from Hawaii to bring news of her sister's death to her parents and to return her husband's ashes to his homeland,[2] the head surgeon at the famous Maeda Clinic[3] recommended Dr. Hayashi's clinic to her when she asked, prompted by an inner voice, if there was any alternative to surgery. He told her that the treatment method used at Dr. Hayashi's clinic was very gentle, so that a "cure" might take weeks or months or even a year. Still, many people were recovering their health through this method.

Takata's own cure required about four months of Reiki treatments at Hayashi's clinic. She felt fascinated by Reiki from the beginning and quickly decided that she wanted to learn for herself how to feel the vibrations that would allow her to sense where there was a need for healing treatment. In this way, she could maintain her own health even after she left Japan.

However, her request was met with initial resistance, for Takata was an "outsider," and unlike all the other practitioners in the clinic, a woman.[4] Eventually, Takata appealed for help to the same surgeon who had recommended Dr. Hayashi's clinic to her in the first place; he wrote a letter to Dr. Hayashi on her behalf requesting that her sincere desire to learn Reiki be given serious consideration. In response, "Dr. Hayashi called the directors of the association to a meeting where

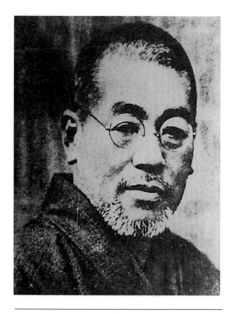

Figure 6.1. Dr. Mikao Usui

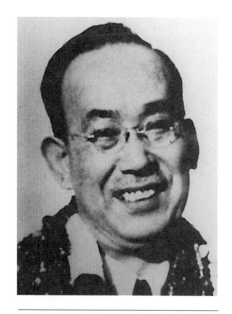

Figure 6.2. Dr. Chujiro Hayashi, Reiki Master, initiated by Dr. Usui

89

this appeal was read. It was decided to allow Takata to become an honorary member, a special privilege which would allow her to take the Reiki lessons. . . ."[5]

Takata learned Reiki at the next opportunity. Dr. Hayashi taught the class over four days, attuning her and her classmates at each class session and providing both practical information on treatment techniques and spiritual instruction. Following the class, Takata became one of the practitioners in Dr. Hayashi's Reiki clinic, assisting in the treatment of patients during the clinic's morning hours and accompanying him on house calls later in the day. This was her work, under his supervision, for the next year. At the end of this apprenticeship, her teacher recognized her dedication to Reiki and rewarded her by permitting her to advance to the next level of training.[6]

When Takata returned home to Hawaii, she did so with the desire to practice Reiki and to establish her own Reiki center. However, she was not yet a teacher. In 1937, Dr. Hayashi and his daughter[7] traveled by sea from Japan to the Territory of Hawaii to visit Takata, to help her introduce Reiki to the public. Dr. Hayashi's free lectures and demonstrations drew crowds, although the trip was not altogether an easy one for him and his daughter. A woman who had begged Takata's help one too many times decided to report the Hayashis to the police, claiming that these "tourists" were charging money for lectures that had been advertised as being free. However, Dr. Hayashi's papers were all in order, and the lectures were indeed free to the public, so the woman's claims were shown to be fraudulent. Hawaiian government officials apologized to the Hayashis, and newspapers reported the story with sympathy, generating even greater interest in Reiki.[8]

Before returning to Japan, Dr. Hayashi, at a banquet in his honor, acknowledged Takata as a Reiki master and recommended her as someone well qualified through her practice and dedication to continue the work he had begun. On February 21, 1938, he certified her as "a practitioner and Master of Dr. Usui's Reiki system of healing." He placed her signed and notarized certificate on file in the offices of the City and County of Honolulu, so that it would be a matter of public record. From that date forward, Takata treated clients and taught Reiki throughout Hawaii.

Before Dr. Hayashi left Hawaii, he asked Takata to come to him again when he sent for her. One year went by, and then another, with no word. Takata

```
                    C E R T I F I C A T E


    THIS IS TO CERTIFY that Mrs. Hawayo Takata, an American
citizen born in the Territory of Hawaii, after a course of study
and training in the Usui system of Reiki healing undertaken
under my personal su-pervision during a visit to Japan in 1935
and subsequently, has passed all the tests and proved worthy and
capable of administering the treatment and of conferring the power
of Reiki on others.
    THEREFORE I, Dr. Chujiro Hayashi, by virtue of my authority as
a Master of the Usui Reiki system of drugless healing, do hereby
confer upon Mrs. Hawayo Takata the full power and authority to
practice the Reiki system and to impart to others the secret
knowledge and the gift of healing under this system.
    MRS. HAWAYO TAKATA is hereby certified by me as a practitioner
and Master of Dr. Usui's Reiki system of healing, at this time
the only person in the United States authorized to confer similar
powers on others and one of the thirteen fully qualified as a
Master of the profession.


    Signed by me the 21st day of February, 1938, in the city and
county of Honolulu, territory of Hawaii.


                                    (SIGNED) Chujiro Hayashi

Witness to his signature:


_____
TERRITORY OF HAWAII,        ⎫
City and County of Honolulu. ⎭ ss.

        On this   21st  day of _____February_____ A.D. 1938   before me
personally appeared
* * * * * * * * (DR.) CHUJIRO HAYASHI* * * * * * * * * * * * * *
to me known to be the person described in and who executed the foregoing
instrument and acknowledged
that  WHO    executed the same as   HIS      free act and deed.

                            _____
                              Notary Public, First Judicial Circuit,
                                 Territory of Hawaii.
ADVERTISER  LEDGER
```

Figure 6.3. *Here is a copy of the text of Hawayo Takata's notarized certificate. Notice that Dr. Hayashi does not use the term "Shinpiden" to describe his own or Takata's level of training. Instead, he translates this term into English, referring to himself as "a Master of the Usui Reiki system of drugless healing" and acknowledging Takata as "one of the thirteen fully qualified as a Master . . ." and "the only person in the United States."*

began to have disturbing dreams about her beloved teacher that aroused her concern.[9] In the dreams, he wore a white ceremonial kimono—associated with death in Japan—and he paced back and forth, hands behind his back, as if anxious about something. Was he dying? Was he ill? She did not know. Was this his way of sending for her, by appearing mysteriously in her dreams? What should she do?

She decided to go to Japan to visit him. In this way, she would see for herself whether all was well. Her trip was quickly arranged. In April 1940, she went to visit Dr. Hayashi at his home. She was pleased that he looked well and this put her mind at ease, but then his wife shared some surprising news with her. Because Japan was on the brink of war with the United States, and Dr. Hayashi was a retired naval officer, he expected that he would be called back to active duty to serve his country once more. Yet in good conscience, he could no longer fight for his country or participate in the violence of the war effort. To do so would violate the principles he lived by as a Buddhist and as a Reiki master. Instead, he would make his transition, a gentle departure from his physical body into eternal life. Although he did not yet know the day and hour, Takata would be invited to be present at that time. Meanwhile, she could journey to the southern part of Japan and learn more about hydrotherapy. When the time came, he would send for her.

A month passed before Takata received word that she was to return to the Hayashi residence in Atami. She traveled all night and arrived early in the morning of May 10th, the day Dr. Hayashi would make his transition. She had the opportunity to talk to him and to learn of his concerns and hopes for the Reiki clinic he had established at Usui's direction in Tokyo. His wife would have to oversee it as well as she was able to during the war, but how successful she would be was uncertain. He encouraged Takata to keep the healing center she had established in Hawaii active and flourishing, despite the coming war. She must safeguard Reiki.

The Hayashis had invited friends and family to gather together to enjoy Dr. Hayashi's company and conversation one last time, at a midday meal. During the meal, Hayashi described to his guests the gentle and painless way in which his transition would occur—three arteries would rupture, one by one, about twenty minutes[10] apart—and it was as he had predicted. Finally, wearing the white silk kimono in which he had appeared in Takata's dreams, he fell backward into the waiting arms of his wife.*

When Takata journeyed home to Hawaii, she had much to reflect on. How could she, someone of Japanese American descent, protect the healing center she had established in Hilo, Hawaii, from the threat of closure and ensure that she herself was regarded as above suspicion? How could she ensure that Reiki survived the coming war? After the bombing of Pearl Harbor on December 7, 1941, Japanese Americans on the mainland were put under surveillance, given curfews, restricted from traveling, and finally forced to evacuate their homes and to report for internment to barracklike camps, guarded by American military personnel. Because Japanese Americans living in the Territory of Hawaii were not regarded as being as dangerous as those on the mainland, they did not suffer these indignities. However, Takata must surely have been sensitive to this atmosphere of suppressed anger and fear. To keep her promise to Dr. Hayashi, she started out by offering treatments and teaching primarily to others of Japanese descent, but she also made some sensible changes, given the political climate: she dropped Japanese language terms; she simplified techniques; she told the story of Mikao Usui in a way that would make it more acceptable to her audience; and in her classes, she insisted that no one take notes.

How did Takata tell the story of Mikao Usui's life and his awakening to

---

*Because Hawayo Takata describes Dr. Hayashi's death from the perspective of an eyewitness, it is important not to discount it, even if her observations are not easily explained or understood in terms of modern medicine. Unfortunately, some modern Reiki masters, unable to make sense of Takata's account, have glossed over the details of the event. Instead, they say, "He took his own life" or even, "He committed suicide." As a result, even some credible sources now describe his death as *seppuku*, or ritual suicide. Others avoid the issue raised by Takata's story of Hayashi's death by saying simply that he ended his life in an honorable way. One Japanese woman has even offered an eyewitness account: Hayashi ran into traffic to save the life of a child. This, too, seems plausible—and certainly more believable than Takata's story.

However, Takata's account is quite detailed. My teacher, Beth Gray, conveyed Takata's sense of awe at witnessing Hayashi's "gentle transition." Why would Takata fabricate such details? Whereas we can understand her embellishment of the story of Mikao Usui's life as evidence of her desire to make the story more acceptable to a Western and primarily Christian audience, no such argument can be made for the account of Hayashi's death. This particular anecdote is not embellished to pleased Westerners or Christians. Instead, we struggle to accept the possibility of his transition taking place as she describes—perhaps in the same way that she herself struggled to accept and understand the event. This story, though we have difficulty comprehending it, has the ring of truth.

Because the luncheon the Hayashi family gave on the day of Dr. Hayashi's death was attended by family members and friends, in time, someone descended from another eyewitness may step forward to offer an account of the same event and validate Takata's observations.

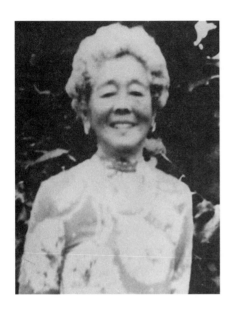

Figure 6.4. *Hawayo Takata, Reiki Master, initiated by Dr. Hayashi*

the healing power of universal life-force energy? Perhaps at first, to other Japanese Americans, she described Mikao Usui simply as a Buddhist who sought enlightenment until one day, after a long meditation, fast, and prayer vigil on Mount Kurama, enlightenment—and empowerment to heal—came to him. However, perhaps even before America declared war on Japan, Takata began to tell the story of Mikao Usui in a way that would make him a more interesting and acceptable "hero" to her Western and primarily Christian audience. A retelling of this story, based on its presentation in Reiki I classes taught by Takata-trained Reiki Master Beth Gray, is included in appendix 1.

Takata repeated her story of Mikao Usui's life and the beginnings of the Reiki system of natural healing many, many times over the more than forty-year span of her career. During the last decade of her life, believing that now she must be the only living Reiki master, Takata decided that she must prepare some of her students to teach Reiki as well—or the method would be lost. She initiated twenty-two people, including my teacher, Reverend Beth Gray, to ensure that Reiki would continue to be taught and practiced.*

---

*The complete list of those who were initiated by Hawayo Takata as Reiki masters, in alphabetical order, is as follows: George Araki; Dorothy Baba; Rick Bockner; Patricia Bowling; Barbara Brown; Fran Brown; Ursula Baylow; Phyllis Lei Furumoto; Beth Gray; John Harvey Gray; Iris Ishikuro; Harry M. Kuboi; Ethel Lombardi; Barbara Lincoln McCullough; Mary McFadyn; Paul Mitchell; Bethel Phaigh; Shinobu Saito; Virginia W. Samdahl; Barbara Weber; and Kay Yamashita.[11]

Even before Takata's death in 1980, these Reiki masters began to teach Usui Shiki Reiki Ryoho around the world, and they told their students the same story of Reiki's beginnings that Takata had told them. They continued to teach Reiki—and students they initiated as Reiki masters have continued to teach Reiki—just as Takata had taught them, passing along this story in each level I class. As a result of their combined efforts, countless millions of people have learned traditional Reiki across the globe and have come to value it for its healing benefits and spiritual comfort.

And now Reiki has found its way to you.

THE RECENT HISTORY OF THE REIKI METHOD

Your teacher may tell you the story of Mikao Usui, as Takata told it, and then perhaps tell her own story of healing and discovery—or she may update Takata's story with information about more recent events, for of course, the history of Reiki did not stop with Takata's initiation of twenty-two Reiki masters to carry on her work.

Here are a few of the events your teacher might mention:

Soon after Takata's death in December 1980, some of her Reiki master students gathered together to discuss how to continue her legacy. A number of these Reiki masters decided to form an organization called the Reiki Alliance and chose Phyllis Furumoto, Takata's granddaughter, to direct the organization. This organization has continued to spread Reiki, largely preserving Takata's way of teaching. However, several of Takata's Reiki master students elected to teach Usui Shiki Ryoho independently (my teacher, Rev. Beth Gray, included), and others went on to teach Reiki under a different name (The Radiance Technique) or in a modified form (Mari-EL).

Takata was interviewed a number of times before her death and articles about her appeared in newspapers and magazines in Hawaii and California. Some of the Reiki masters she initiated were also interviewed in the 1970s and 1980s, and the articles written about them helped to attract students to their classes. In the early 1980s, the first books about Reiki began to appear on bookstore shelves, a departure from the "oral tradition" Takata had proclaimed as the primary method of teaching. One of the earliest of these books, *The Reiki Handbook: A Manual for Students and Therapists of the Usui Shiki Ryoho System of Healing*,[12] based on instruction provided by Takata-trained Reiki Master Virginia Samdahl, provided photographs of hand positions to be used for self-treatment and for client treatment; recounted the story of Dr. Usui; and recommended certain hand positions for treatment of specific conditions.

Another book, Diane Stein's *Essential Reiki*,[13] presented the author's unorthodox journey to Reiki mastery, and then offered another set of hand positions for self treatment and client treatment, many variations of the symbols typically learned in a Reiki II class, and even variations of the master symbol. Since Takata had demanded secrecy regarding the symbols, this book caused great controversy. The ensuing dialogue was healthy, for it helped traditionally taught practitioners and teachers understand that Takata did not always teach Reiki I and II in the same way. If hand positions, symbols, and even distant-healing methods could vary, then the essence of Reiki was not contained in any one form.* Truly, the essence of Reiki is universal life-force energy itself, something Takata knew well—and trusted—as she taught her students based on her own evolving understanding and her present-moment inner guidance.

The dissemination of information about Reiki, in English and other languages, in books and articles, continued as it became more widely known around the world for its effectiveness in healing. It was only a matter of time before someone would go to Japan to research the origins of Reiki. Frank Arjava Petter, who learned Reiki in Germany in 1992, moved to Japan in 1993 and began to teach there, only to discover that some of his students were already familiar with the energy work he taught. Through one of his students, he made contact with an individual named Mr. Tsutomu Oishi,[15] who had learned Reiki from Mr. Kozo Ogawa, who claimed to have been made a teacher by Mikao Usui. Mr. Oishi described Mr. Ogawa's Reiki center in Shizuoka, provided a new photograph of Mikao Usui, and suggested where Petter should continue his research.

In 1997, Frank Arjava Petter's book, *Reiki Fire: New Information about the Origins of the Reiki Power,* was published in German and English. This book included a new photo of Mikao Usui (given to Petter by Mr. Oishi[16]), and mul-

---

*Writes Helen J. Haberly, "Specific hand positions are taught for the sake of expedience since long practice has shown these to work efficiently; however, there is no 'wrong' way to do Reiki—and, thus, no 'right' way."[14]

tiple photos of Mikao Usui's gravesite and the Usui Memorial, a tall stone that stands beside it, in the cemetery of Saihoji Temple in Tokyo.[17] The photo of Mikao Usui was "captioned" by bold, black strokes of Japanese calligraphy, which proved to be the Gainen, the more complete text of the Reiki principles. Petter's translation of the Usui Memorial also featured the Gainen, making the significance of these guidelines for daily life even clearer.

Here is a translation of the complete inscription on the Usui Memorial, provided by Rev. Hyakuten Inamoto and reprinted with his kind permission.[18] Your Reiki master is welcome to read the text aloud to you in class to give you another perspective on Reiki's early history:

That which is attained within oneself after having accumulated the fruits of disciplined study and training is called "Toku" and that which can be offered to others after having spread a path of teaching and salvation is called "Koh." Only with high merits and great virtues can one be a great founding teacher. Sagacious and brilliant men of the olden time or the founders of new teachings and religious sects were all like that. Someone like Usui Sensei can be counted among them. Sensei newly founded the method based on Reiki of the universe to improve the mind and body. Having heard of his reputation all over, people crowded around to seek his teachings and treatments. Ah, how popular it is!

Sensei, commonly known by the name 'Mikao,' with an extra name (pseudonym) 'Gyohan' was from Taniai-mura (village), Yamagata-gun (county), Gifu-ken (prefecture). He is descended from Chiba Tsunetane. His father's name was Taneuji, and was commonly called Uzaemon. His mother was from the Kawai family.

Sensei was born on August 15 of the first year of Keio (A.D. 1865). From his youth he surpassed his fellows in hard work and endeavor. When he grew up he visited Europe and America, and studied in China. Despite his will to succeed in life, he was stalemated and fell into great difficulties. However, in the face of adversity he strove to train himself even more with the courage never to yield.

One day, he climbed Kurama-yama and after twenty-one days of a severe discipline without eating, he suddenly felt One Great Reiki over his head and attained enlightenment and he obtained Reiki Ryoho. Then, he tried

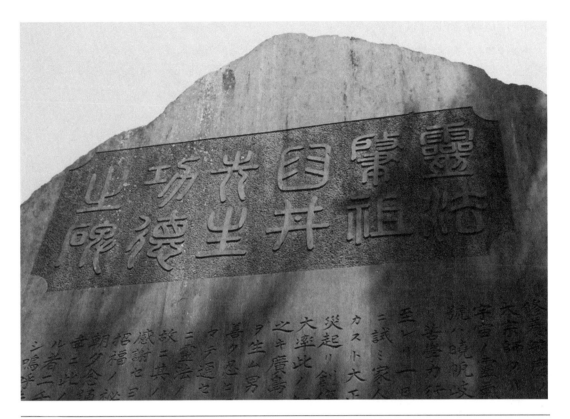

Figure 6.5. *These Japanese characters at the very top of the Usui Memorial read: "Reiho Choso Usui Sensei Kudoku No Hi," which translates into English as "Memorial of the merits of Usui Sensei, the founder of Reiho" (Reiki Ryoho).*

it on himself and experimented on his family members. The efficacy was immediate. Sensei thought that it would be far better to offer it widely to the general public and share its benefits than just to improve the well-being of his own family members.

In April of the 11th year of Taisho (A.D. 1922) he settled in Harajuku, Aoyamo, Tokyo and set up the Gakkai to teach Reiki Ryoho and give treatments. Even outside of the building it was full of pairs of shoes of the visitors who had come from far and near.

In September of the 12th year (A.D. 1923) there was a great earthquake and a conflagration broke out. Everywhere there were groans of pain from the wounded. Sensei, feeling pity for them, went out every morning to go around the town, and he cured and saved innumerable people. This is just a broad outline of his relief activities during such an emergency.

Later on, as the 'dojo' became too small, in February of the 14th year (A.D. 1925) the new suburban house was built at Nakano according to divination. Due to his respected and far-reaching reputation many people from local districts wished to invite him. Sensei, accepting the invitations, went to Kure and then to Hiroshima and Saga, and reached Fukuyama. Unexpectedly he became ill and passed away there. It was March 9 of the 15th year of Taisho (A.D. 1926), [he was] aged 62.

His spouse was Suzuki, and was called Sadako. One boy and one girl were born. The boy was named Fuji and he succeeded to the family. Sensei's personality was gentle and modest and he never behaved ostentatiously. His physique was large and sturdy. He always wore a contented smile. He was stout-hearted, tolerant and very prudent upon undertaking a task. He was by nature versatile and loved to read books. He engaged himself in history books, medical books, Buddhist scriptures, Christian scriptures and was well versed in psychology, Taoism, even in the art of divination, incantation, and physiognomy. Presumably Sensei's background in the arts and sciences afforded him nourishment for his cultivation and discipline, and it was very obvious that it was this cultivation and discipline that became the key to the creation of Reiho (Reiki Ryoho).

On reflection, Reiho puts special emphasis not just on curing diseases but also on enjoying wellbeing in life with correcting the mind and making the body healthy with the use of an innate healing ability. Thus, before teaching, the 'Ikun' (admonition) of the Meiji Emperor should reverently be read and Five Precepts be chanted and kept in mind mornings and evenings.

Firstly it reads, 'Today do not anger,' secondly it reads, 'Do not worry,' thirdly it reads 'Be thankful,' fourthly it reads, 'Work with diligence,' fifthly it reads, 'Be kind to others.'

These are truly great teachings for cultivation and discipline that agree with those great teachings of the ancient sages and the wise. Sensei named these teachings 'Secret Method to Invite Happiness' and 'Miraculous Medicine to Cure All Diseases.' Notice the outstanding features of the teachings. Furthermore, when it comes to teaching, it should be as easy and common as possible, nothing lofty.

Another noted feature is that during sitting in silent meditation with Gassho and reciting the Five Precepts mornings and evenings, the pure and healthy mind can be cultivated and put into practice in one's daily routine. This is the reason why Reiho is easily obtained by anyone.

Recently the course of the world has shifted and a great change in thought has taken place. Fortunately with the spread of this Reiho, there will be many that supplement the way of the world and the minds of people. How can it be for just the benefit of curing chronic diseases and longstanding complaints?

A little more than 2,000 people became students of Sensei. Those senior disciples living in Tokyo gathered at the dojo and carried on the work (of the late Sensei) and those who lived in local districts also spread the teachings. Although Sensei is gone, Reiho should still be widely propagated in the world for a long time. Ah, how prominent and great Sensei is that he offers the teachings to people out there after having been enlightened within!

Of late the fellow disciples consulted with each other about building the stone memorial in the graveyard of Saihoji Temple in Toyotama-gun so as to honor his merits and to make them immortalized and I was asked to write it.

As I deeply submit to Sensei's greatness and am happy for the very friendly teacher-disciple relationships among fellow students, I could not decline the request, and I wrote a summary in the hope that people in the future shall be reminded to look up at him in reverence.

February, the 2nd year of Showa (A.D. 1927)
Composed by: Okada Masayuki, Doctor of Literature
                Ju-sanmi (subordinate 3rd rank),
                Kun-santo (the 3rd Order of Merit)
Calligraphy by: Ushida Juzabura, Navy Rear Admiral
                Ju-yonmi (subordinate 4th rank),
                Kun-santo (the 3rd Order of Merit)
                Ko-yonkyu (the distinguished service 4th class)

In 1998, Frank Arjava Petter published a second ground-breaking book, *Reiki: The Legacy of Dr. Usui,* which featured a new, more complete translation

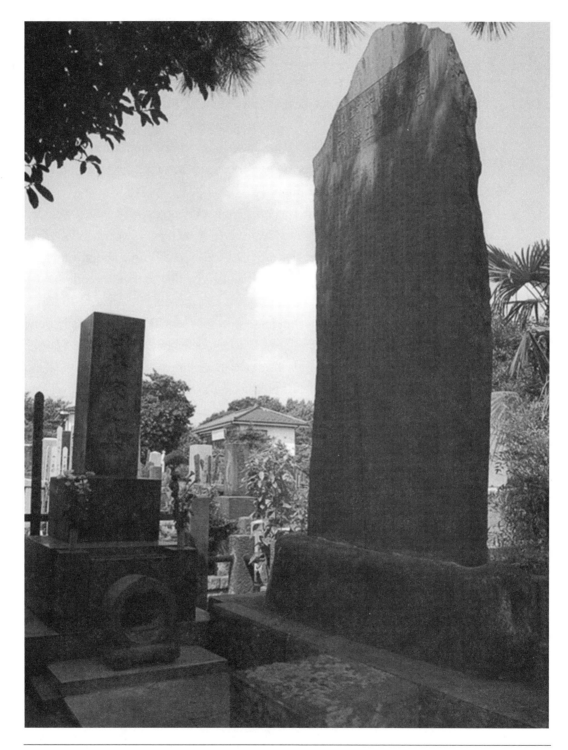

Figure 6.6. *The Usui Memorial, beside the gravesite of Mikao Usui, is an eloquent testimony to the love and respect that his students and his patients felt for him.*

of the Reiki principles and also parts of the *Reiki Ryoho Hikkei* (handbook), which Dr. Usui gave to his beginner students. Here were Dr. Usui's explanation of Reiki, his answers to some frequently asked questions, some recommended hand positions for certain medical conditions, and 125 poems (waka) written by the Meiji Emporer that Dr. Usui found to contain some spiritual wisdom. The same year, Mr. Hiroshi Doi, a Japanese Reiki master and a member of the Reiki Ryoho Gakkai, kindly accepted an invitation to visit the West and share information about Reiki's early history.

In August 1999, before an international group of Reiki masters, which included both Frank Arjava Petter and Wanja Twan, one of the twenty-two Reiki masters trained by Hawayo Takata, Mr. Doi provided still more details about the life of Mikao Usui and the learning society he founded, which still exists today. With the knowledge and permission of the current chairperson, he described historically based Usui Reiki Ryoho techniques, some of them similar and many quite different from the techniques taught in Usui Shiki Ryoho classes in the West.

Over the next several years, Mr. Doi, often accompanied by his good friend and fellow Reiki master, Rev. Hyakuten Inamoto, has continued to travel and to share knowledge of Reiki's early history, teaching methods, and techniques; he also teaches Gendai Reiki, his synthesis of traditional Japanese and Western Reiki techniques. Rev. Inamoto teaches Komyo Reiki, another synthesis of traditional Japanese and Western Reiki based on his training with Mrs. Chiyoko Yamaguchi (now deceased), a Second Degree student of Dr. Chujiro Hayashi raised to the Shihan or teacher level by Wasaburo Sagano, her uncle, who (like Hawayo Takata) was initiated as a Shinpiden by Dr. Hayashi. Tadao Yamaguchi, Mrs. Yamaguchi's son, also travels outside Japan, teaching Jikiden Reiki, following the manner of Hayashi.[19]

The result of all this cultural exchange is a tremendous opportunity for healing. Those who have been taught Usui Shiki Reiki Ryoho by their Takata-trained Reiki masters have an opportunity to listen with an open mind to the information that has been so generously offered. We now may appreciate Mikao Usui in a new way, meditate upon the original Reiki principles he adopted with deeper understanding, and consider the explanations of the Reiki method that he offered in his manual, the *Usui Reiki Hikkei,* with greater attention to the universal truths he expresses.

THE SOURCE OF REIKI ENERGY

It is our own awakening to the Reiki energy that can enable us to see beyond the words of one story or another about its history to its true essence. "Our Reiki Ryoho is something absolutely original and cannot be compared with any other (spiritual) path in the world," Mikao Usui wrote in the *Reiki Ryoho Hikkei*.[20] "This is why I would like to make this method (freely) available to the public for the well-being of humanity. Each of us has the potential of being given a gift by the divine, which results in the body and soul becoming unified. In this way (with Reiki), a great many people will experience the blessing of the divine . . . our Reiki Ryoho is an original therapy, which is built upon the spiritual power of the universe."[21]

In her early diary, Takata writes, "I believe there exists One Supreme Being—the Absolute Infinite—a Dynamic Force that governs the world and universe. It is an unseen spiritual power that vibrates and all other powers fade into insignificance beside it. So, therefore, it is Absolute!

"This power is unfathomable, immeasurable, and being a universal life force, it is incomprehensible to man. . . . I shall call it 'Reiki' because I studied under that expression. . . . Reiki . . . comes from the Great Spirit, the Infinite."[22]

When we consider the origin of Reiki, it might be well to remember that the origin of the universe and of life itself have been debated by philosophers and religious teachers throughout recorded history. Modern science offers multiple theories, yet no one can say for certain: this is how the universe came into being; this is how it will end. The practice of Reiki gradually teaches us something that might otherwise be considered unknowable: each time we use our hands to offer healing, we experience a flow of healing energy from an infinite source, and that flow is apparently guided by a greater intelligence than our own—higher, wiser, and more compassionate.

If Reiki is the answer to Mikao Usui's question, what was that question? What is the purpose of life? What is the nature of healing? What is the source of healing? How is it possible to experience enlightenment? What does it mean to be happy? Let the stories of Reiki's early history help you to understand that others before you have been challenged to search for answers to such spiritual questions—and have found them in Reiki. May you also find the answers that you seek.

7

A METAPHYSICAL
APPROACH TO HEALING,
HEALTH, AND WELLNESS

The word *origin* can mean beginning, source, or cause. When we reflect on the origin of Reiki healing, we can think in terms of history, religion and spirituality, philosophy, or science. When was Reiki first taught and practiced? What is the origin of universal life-force energy? Does healing become more complete and lasting when the cause of poor health is understood? How does Reiki restore the physical body to natural balance? All of these questions are worthy of serious consideration—and the answers are not all in.

Yet even without having all the answers, Reiki practitioners, for generations, have successfully treated countless people worldwide—and many of those people have become practitioners as well, simply because "Reiki works." Sometimes immediate, dramatic healing occurs. At other times, pain is relieved and symptoms improved during the first Reiki treatment but the benefits continue to accrue with subsequent treatments. Is there anything practitioners or clients can do to speed healing, besides simply being open to receive the Reiki energy? As it turns out, there is something we can do—and that is to come to a more conscious understanding of the intimate relationship between the body and the mind. What causes sickness? What triggers pain? What changes the signs of prolonged tension and stress into the symptoms of a chronic medical condition? How is it that our emotional and mental response to loss or trauma can lower our immune system defenses and make us more vulnerable to accidental injury, acute illness, or even life-threatening disease?

Hawayo Takata often said, "Find the cause and you will remove the effect. . . . Only when the cause is removed will the benefit of treatment be long lasting."[1] My forward-thinking Reiki teacher, Beth Gray, accepted this idea as well, and she made it clear that she believed the "cause" of the "effect" of physical illness was often emotional or mental in nature. What she called our "stinking thinking" could set us up for "issues in the tissues."[2] When an emotional upset leaves us feeling that we cannot let go of anger or worry, or disappointment or loss triggers depression that we cannot shake, we do become more prone to accidental injury and to acute illness. When negative thoughts and feelings become habitual, the risk of serious illness rises.

Recent research supports this holistic view. Not only has quantum physics given us a new understanding of the relationship of thought to energy and matter, but molecular and behavioral neuroscientists have determined that the chemical receptors that mediate emotion are present in the brain and in the tissues of the immune system—bone marrow, thymus, spleen, lymph nodes and vessels. This directly links the power of a patient's thoughts and feelings to his ability to fight disease.

Although most people find that this new vision of the mind and body feels right, when I first learned Reiki in 1987, I felt very uncomfortable with the ease with which my fellow students and practitioners told tales about the dangers of negative thinking and suppressed emotion. I fidgeted in my seat as I listened to stories like these:

> "My friend John had a heart attack and died just six months after his wife. He was really close to her. He told me at his wife's funeral that he didn't know what he was going to do without her. He said she had been his reason for living."
>
> "My sister-in-law has known that her husband was having an affair for years, and

it has just been eating away at her inside. Now she has been diagnosed with breast cancer."

I felt frightened by the implication that negative thoughts and feelings might eventually be expressed in the body as disease. Was every dark and idle thought so dangerous? Did every blue day become translated into the physical body as aches and pains? The consequences of being "free thinking" seemed grave, and the task of controlling conscious mind looked overwhelming.

The class discussion turned toward solutions. The cautionary words of Peter McWilliams in *You Can't Afford the Luxury of a Negative Thought* were brought up, as well as Alice Steadman's *Who's the Matter With Me?*[3] The power of positive thinking was described, and the use of affirmations recommended, particularly for transforming negative thoughts about illness and pain into habitual positive thoughts with beneficial effects. My teacher praised the work of Louise L. Hay, who had cured herself of cancer after being told she was terminally ill; her books, especially *You Can Heal Your Life,*[4] were recommended. Clearly, my teacher believed Hay's message that "The thoughts you choose to think create the experiences you have."[5]

I wasn't satisfied. Even as a child, I had struggled to understand how to control my conscious mind. As an adult who sat in daily meditation, I still struggled—and tried not to struggle. I wasn't happy being told to "do the mental work." I felt more deeply moved—and changed in consciousness—by my teacher's four guided meditations, on love, gratitude, forgiveness, and joy. These evoked a sense of connection to Spirit, quieting my mind and calming my physical body, which recommendations to practice positive thinking did not.

During the years that followed, I did learn to use affirmations to change my mood and to create a reality that was more in line with what I wanted. I also used visualization, prayer, and meditation to focus my intentions, ask for guidance, and center and calm my mind. All were effective—but none seemed to be as enduringly effective in changing my thoughts and feelings as simply practicing Reiki. For this reason, I found it difficult to make a daily habit of the affirmations and visualizations; prayer was already a habit. And Reiki? Reiki simply flowed through my hands with the energy of unconditional love, whether I was thinking positively or not, whether I was distracted or distressed or not. The experience of Reiki was so forgiving of my restless mind that I fell in love with it and have remained in love ever since.

I know now that I missed part of Louise Hay's message, as we talked about her work in class: "When a client comes to me, no matter how dire their predicament seems to be, I *know* if they are *willing* to do the mental work of releasing and forgiving, almost anything can be healed. The word 'incurable' which is so frightening to so many people, really only means that the particular condition cannot be cured by 'outer' methods and that we must *go within* to effect the healing."[6] The mental work recommended to us in class is not simply a matter of changing negative thought patterns. To create permanent healing it is necessary to change the mind. To change the mind, it is necessary to change the heart.

Research in psychoneuroimmunology—the study of how mind and body affect the immune system—supports this. Using MRI and CAT scan technologies, scientists are able to watch the brain as a person thinks and feels. The cerebral cortex, the most recently evolved part of the brain, sparks with the movement of a single thought. The amygdala, in the much older mid-brain, lights with emotion. This research and related work with brain-injured patients has led scientists to understand that "the amygdala has a greater capacity to control the cortex than the cortex to control the amygdala."[7] In other words, emotions rule thoughts, rather than the other way around. Or, as poet e.e. cummings wrote, "Feeling is first."[8] This may be one of the reasons that Reiki is so transforming, healing the practitioner as well as the client over time on all levels of being. Love rules. Unconditional love rules with an even stronger hand.

All traditional Usui Reiki attunements open energy centers at the crown of the head, the heart, and the hands to the flow of life-force energy. (In one Reiki class at which I assisted, Reiki Master Beth Gray showed us a photograph of one of her students who had just received an attunement. A wide, white ray of light radiated from above toward the student's heart. In photo after photo, the ray remained focused on the student's heart. It was not a trick, not retouched, not a problem on the film; what is usually invisible simply had been made visible.) Besides opening the energy centers to allow practitioners to channel Reiki healing energy, the attunements also bring healing to the mind, the heart, and the body; practitioners often remark that they feel a comforting sense of peace, a gentle compassion, or unconditional love.

Studies at the Institute of HeartMath in Boulder Creek, California, have demonstrated "that our positive emotions can change the energy field surrounding our hearts. If we feel, flowing through our heart, joy or love for someone or compassion for the helpless, our heartbeat becomes more regular." Furthermore, the heart will "pull, or entrain, other organs in the body into the same rhythm," including the brain. The result is that "if the heartbeat is regular, it brings corresponding increases in clarity, buoyancy, intuitive awareness, and peacefulness," as well as improved health and stronger immune system response.[9]

While I cannot say with certainty that my heartbeat is more regular when I am doing Reiki, I can say that the sense of compassion that I feel that begins in my heart soon encompasses my whole being, and that this experience is common to practitioners. With the love for life and the compassion that we feel as we practice, we can "entrain" our conscious thoughts more easily, make affirmations with stronger conviction, visualize with greater clarity, and pray with sincere gratitude. In this gentle and indirect way, we can work with Reiki's subtle energy to heal our own negativity.

SPECIFIC TECHNIQUES FOR MENTAL AND EMOTIONAL HEALING

Even with training only in Reiki hands-on healing, there are some specific hand positions that you, as a practitioner, can use to cope with stress, ease tension, relieve anxious thoughts, and calm turbulent emotions. When you apply Reiki using these hand positions, you do intervention. How can this be so effective? When you recognize your feelings of distress in response to a difficult situation and you immediately use Reiki, the energy flow quickly relaxes you and eases your tension. The result is that you are more quickly able to recover your composure and positive attitude, remember your problem-solving skills, and take any appropriate action. And as you consistently use these positions, day by day, to maintain emotional balance and peace of mind, you may find that depression dissipates, blue moods brighten, and negative thoughts stop taking hold.

Some of the positions recommended below are included in the standard treatment of the abdomen, the head, and the back. However, many practitioners find them useful to "Band-Aid" the physical body and the energy field during the day to calm turbulent emotions and confused thoughts. Other suggested hand positions will be new to you. Use whatever positions seem most helpful—and feel free to use your hands to deliver Reiki to yourself wherever you personally manifest symptoms triggered by stress. For example, if you are an asthma sufferer, use your Reiki-charged hands on your upper chest area whenever you feel your breathing start to tighten; if you have a history of panic attacks, use your hands over your heart to slow its racing, at your upper midriff (over the adrenal glands) to recover calm, and in any and all head positions that seem appropriate to bring your anxious mind to the recognition that all is well. Do your best to remain comfortable as you move from position to position, or you will be less effective in delivering the treatment.

Taming Tension Headaches and Migraines (Figure 7.1)

When you feel a headache beginning, you can use Reiki to stop it from becoming full-fledged. Simply place one hand across your forehead, at about the level of the hairline, and the other across the back of your head, so that it covers the base of the skull, just above the cervical vertebrae of the neck. Feel the flow of Reiki energy and marvel at how quickly your headache disappears. Most tension headaches can be successfully treated within a couple minutes.

If the headache seems to be triggered by eyestrain, do an extra position over your eyes (Basic II, position 1)—and be kind to your body! Turn off the computer, close the book, get some sleep, or even invest in a new pair of eyeglasses.

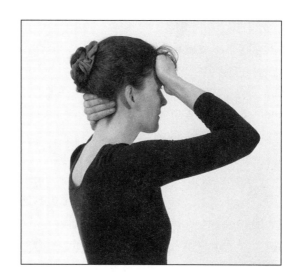

Figure 7.1. A Reiki-charged hand on the forehead and one at the base of the skull will usually alleviate a tension headache quickly.

Do whatever is necessary to take better care of yourself; in this way, you can maintain the health that Reiki has enabled you to reclaim and build an even stronger sense of well-being.

Migraine sufferers will need to do more positions, both hands on and in the energy field, to dissipate the aura that precedes a migraine or to reduce the pain of a migraine that is already in progress. If you have developed sufficient sensitivity in your hands (which comes soon with daily practice), slowly move your hands around the head, front and back and sides, to scan it and to determine where healing is needed. Wherever your hands turn on, apply your Reiki-charged hands to the corresponding physical area and in the energy field above it. Be thorough. Listen to your hands in each position and allow them to remain in place through a complete cycle of the energy flow.

Remember, too, that besides being caused by stress, migraines can be triggered by other causes, including allergies, hormonal imbalances, and the weather. While you can't necessarily do much about the weather, you can apply your hands to your stomach if you are reacting to something you ate and to your head and abdomen if you are suffering from hormonal imbalance. Because the causes of a migraine are often complex, successful treatment may take some time. You may be able to dissipate a pre-migraine aura in twenty minutes or so, but if a migraine has taken hold, be prepared to treat yourself for an hour or more to make it manageable.

Facing Off Frustration (Figure 7.2)

If you are someone who often suppresses annoyance, frustration, or anger on the job or at home, you may find yourself clenching your jaw throughout the day or grinding your teeth at night. The resulting face ache, often focused in the TMJ (tempo-mandibular joint) can be debilitating. As you live through the moment of near confrontation, make an effort to focus on your breathing. As you inhale, consciously breathe in more deeply and slowly, and as you exhale, feel your shoulders relax and deliberately let the negative thoughts and feelings go. Remember the first Reiki principle: "Just for today, do not anger . . ."

As soon as you have the opportunity to be alone, in your cubicle or in your kitchen, lean on your desk top or kitchen table and support your head in your hands. With your wrists meeting under your chin, your palms covering your lower face, and your fingertips touching the tempo-mandibular joint, the flow of Reiki will relieve the physical tension and calm disturbed emotions and disordered thoughts.

Just Don't Want to Hear It? (Figure 7.3)

The mind-body may manifest earache, ear infections, and even temporary or permanent loss of hearing in response to stressful words and disturbing conversations; it is not only ongoing noise pollution or sharp or high decibel noises that put people at risk.

If you find that you have been tuning out a conversation that is too painful to hear, please take the time soon afterward to use your Reiki-charged hands on your ears. Simply cover your ears with your hands, as if you "just don't want to hear it." Enjoy the healing energy flow and let the anxious feelings go. Allow the Reiki energy to quiet your mind's comments about what has taken place. Remember the second Reiki principle, "Just for today, do not worry . . ."

**Maintaining Peace of Mind:
The Chalice (Figure 7.4)**

How very precious is peace of mind! And what a challenge it can be to maintain mental tranquility through the day, when any unplanned event can cause a delay in a tightly planned schedule. A suit jacket has a stain on the lapel. A tire is flat. Road construction delays your arrival time. A train is late. A coworker cannot make a meeting. A proposal is not approved. A budget must be reworked. Your spouse can't pick up the kids after school. The babysitter isn't available. The power goes out during the night and you wake to the alarm clock flashing 12:00 over and over again. When such

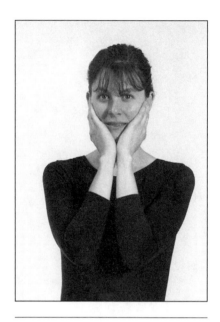

Figure 7.2. Place your hands over your jaw if you find yourself gritting your teeth in annoyance during the day or grinding them in suppressed frustration in your sleep at night.

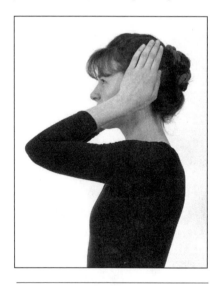

Figure 7.3. Protect your future hearing by using this position after an argument.

111

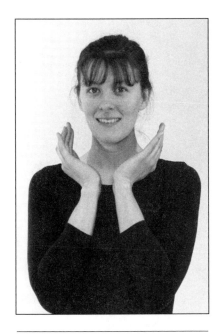

Figure 7.4. Comfort yourself and protect your peace of mind by using your hands as shown.

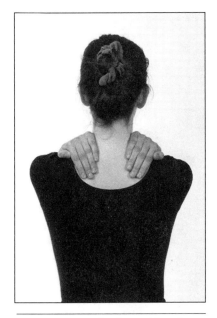

Figure 7.5. Reiki-charged hands can soothe tense shoulders and upper back.

small mishaps can throw you off balance, how do you manage when real disaster occurs?

"The Chalice" can help. Hold your hands in the energy field, a few inches under your chin and throat, as if you were cradling a light and wanted to protect it from wind and sleet and snow. You will be directing energy into the mid-brain cavity through the soft tissues of your chin and throat; the energy will also penetrate the bones of the jaw, as well as the sinuses at the back of the nose and behind the eye sockets. This position is very soothing—and it is an excellent position to use when you want to protect your entire body from the effects of daily stress or shock in response to disaster: hands applied here support the health of all the endocrine system glands housed in the mid-brain cavity, including the hypothalamus, which mediates the response to stress in every cell.

Shrugging Off Shoulder Tension (Figure 7.5)
Sometimes, when you feel tied to your desk for too many hours on end, the stress of the long day can result in contracted muscles in your shoulders. On arrival home, even the clatter of pots and pans in the kitchen or the noise of the phone ringing can send another jolt of tension through you, tightening the knots in your shoulders even more.

Treat yourself to a hot shower when you can, but for now, reach for your shoulders with your Reiki-charged hands and let the energy begin to relax the physical tension that has built up there. As you listen to the energy, shrug your shoulders, roll your neck—and breathe. You can cooperate with the healing that is occurring on all levels by consciously choosing to remember the third Reiki principle: "Be grateful." When you begin to count your blessings, you will discover that it is easier to shift your attention away from the difficulties of the day that is past to the simple pleasures present at this moment.

Healing Heartache (Figure 7.6)

Sometimes people are surprised to discover that emotional disappointment or loss can result in a feeling of heartache or heartbreak that feels so physically real. Sadly, if this unhappiness is not addressed, years of sustained heartache can eventually manifest in the physical body as heart disease or heart attack.

As preventive energy medicine, when you experience an emotional loss, treat your heart with the flow of unconditional love through your Reiki-attuned hands. When a friend disappoints you, when a loved one forgets a birthday, when someone you love leaves you, no matter what the reason, take time—repeatedly—to treat your heart until you again feel well. If you follow your hands-on treatment of your heart with work in your energy field, a few inches away from the body, in the area that Indian yogis call the "heart chakra," you will feel even more comforted and soothed, for you will be healing your energy field, which may be weakened by your loss. Your energy field can also hold potential problems not yet manifested in the physical body, as well as habitual thoughts and feelings. Reiki applied here brings healing to you now and helps to assure a healthier future.

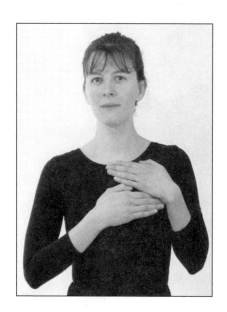

Figure 7.6. Use your Reiki-attuned hands over your heart to heal heartache as well as any physical weakness or heart condition.

If you are a new practitioner and you don't feel the subtle flow of Reiki healing as clearly when you work in the energy field as you do when you work with your hands on the body, just be patient. Continue to treat yourself daily with Reiki. As long as you are consistent in your practice, this awareness will eventually come. It might take a couple months. It might take six months or even more. (You can test your own sensitivity to the energy field periodically by slowly scanning the front of your body along the centerline, from the top of your head to the base of the spine. The seven major chakras—crown, third eye, throat, heart, solar plexus, sacrum, and root—are usually the most pronounced features of the energy field and the easiest to notice as your sensitivity increases.)

But if you don't sense the flow of the energy to the chakras within the first few months of learning Reiki, don't worry about it. Continue to treat yourself with the standard positions and any extra positions that feel appropriate. Remember the fourth Reiki principle, sometimes translated this way: "Do your best."

Healing the "Fight or Flight" Response (Figure 7.7 and Figure 7.8)

Everyone is familiar with the rush of adrenaline shooting through the bloodstream in response to danger, and some people even seek it out, deliberately

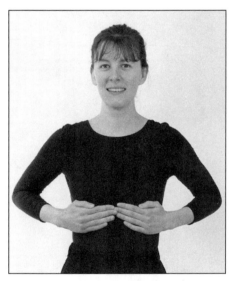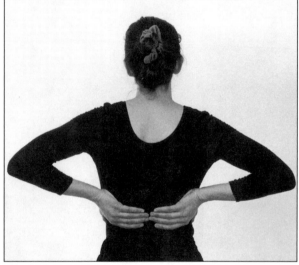

Figures 7.7 and 7.8. *Quiet the rush of adrenaline by using your Reiki-charged hands over your midriff, in Basic I, position 1, or over your mid-back, in Basic III, position 1.*

choosing high risk occupations or hobbies in order to satisfy the need for this natural "high." However, most people find the sensation of readiness for fight or flight uncomfortable—and our fast-paced, high-tech culture promotes a constant readiness, which can exhaust the adrenals and make us feel worn out.

The adrenal glands are located under the muscles and ribs of the mid-back; they literally sit atop the renal organs—the kidneys. If you are committed to your practice, and you treat yourself each day, you will find your hands in the appropriate position (Basic I, position 1 or Basic III, position 1) to support your adrenal glands at least once a day. This will gradually restore your sense of calm and readiness to cope with emergencies if you have been under stress for a long time. If you find yourself dealing with a crisis, however, take the time to focus on your adrenals as soon as your hands are free. Although you may have other areas of injury that you want to treat first, placing your hands over your midriff or over your mid-back area to support the adrenals can help you avoid slipping into shock or help you to recover from it more quickly.

Feeling Manipulated? Focus on the Solar Plexus (Figure 7.9)

In Indian yoga, the solar plexus chakra, which is located at mid-body, around the navel, is regarded as having to do with the exercise of free will and with emotions. So if you feel that your good ideas are being ignored or your creativity

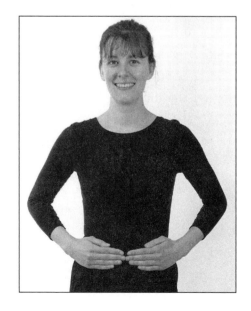

Figure 7.9. The Basic I, position 3 hand position, over the solar plexus chakra, can be used anytime during the day that you feel yourself being pushed or pulled at by people and circumstances; it is calming.

is not being allowed adequate expression, you may feel a corresponding physical discomfort here—"knots" in the stomach, nausea, a feeling of having been punched in the stomach, or something similar.

Attend to this emotional disquiet and mental discord by placing your hands over the middle of your abdomen at the level of the navel. Again, if you treat yourself daily with the standard hand positions for Basic I, you will usually find that you are able to take life's small blows with calm, but if something occurs that triggers an upset stomach or a feeling of coldness in the pit of your stomach, take the time immediately or as soon as possible to "Band-Aid" this area. You will not only be addressing the physical effect, but the emotional and mental cause. And if you do not have both hands free, then use just one hand. You will discover that relief is almost immediate with the application of Reiki.

Combining Positions

Emotions are often complex. We may feel grief, disappointment, and anxiety all at the same time; we may feel sadness and gladness at once. When you find yourself responding to an upsetting situation with a tapestry of emotions rather than a single thread of feeling, use your Reiki-charged hands to calm your mind, ease heartache, and settle your stomach.

Here is a story to illustrate the value of using combined positions:

One autumn day in 2003, I went to the hospital to visit my elderly mother, only to discover that the doctor most recently assigned to her case had passed it off to another doctor who hadn't even reviewed her chart; he knew absolutely nothing about her undiagnosed illness or its treatment to date. When I met him for the first time in the corridor outside my mother's room, he couldn't answer a single question or respond to any concerns.

I heard myself raising my voice to him—something I rarely do, as I am not given to anger. I stopped myself, turned on my heel, and walked away from him as fast as I could. I raced across the parking lot, opened my locked car door, slid in behind the wheel, and realized that I was in no shape to drive. I was angry, frustrated, filled with adrenaline, and grieving over my mother's suffering.

I sat still. I slowed my breath. I put one hand over my heart and the other over my solar plexus. The Reiki energy coursed into me, and I began to feel calmer. I stayed in that position for perhaps ten minutes, and then I moved my hands, still at heart and solar plexus level, into my energy field. I felt the energy hum around my body, restoring me to harmony and balance. I remained in this position, comforted by the flow of Reiki from my hands into my entire energy field, for another ten minutes or so.

Finally, I searched for my keys in my purse, put the car key in the ignition, and started the car. I knew that I could drive safely—and I knew that I had to accept with serenity a situation that I could not change. And somehow, if I could, I had to reach deeply enough within to remember the fifth Reiki principle, "Be kind." The next time that I saw this physician, I had to find a way to be considerate and warm to him if I wanted him to give greater consideration to my mother.

THE REIKI PRINCIPLES

Your traditional Reiki teacher may present the Reiki principles to you as part of Hawayo Takata's story or as part of the inscription on the Usui Memorial. Takata taught them to her students in slightly different versions, encouraging the students to regard them as ideals for daily life. My teacher, Rev. Beth Gray, presented them as follows:

> *Just for today, do not worry.*
> *Just for today, do not anger.*
> *Just for today, be grateful for all life's blessings.*
> *Just for today, do an honest day's work.*
> *Just for today, be kind to every living thing.*

These statements are not commandments that must be obeyed. They are not "dogma" or church doctrine that must be believed. They are principles that embody values, which, if practiced, help us lead healthy lives: acceptance, peace of mind, gratitude, integrity, kindness and compassion. If we treat the Reiki principles as mental touchstones throughout the day, whenever circumstances tempt us to worry or to be anxious, to bridle or to complain or to resent, we discover that our attitudes subtly change. The stress-causing negative thoughts and feelings are displaced and dissolved by the power of positive thoughts and

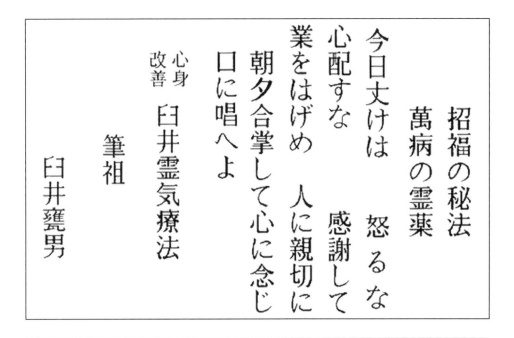

Figure 7.10. The Gainen, the complete Reiki principles, with Mikao Usui's double titles and recommendation to do meditation, are read from right to left and top to bottom; see if you can discern the orderly arrangement of the modern Japanese kanji in this image of the Gainen, created on a personal computer.

feelings. This is another step toward complete self-healing, consciously chosen; this is a change in our minds that supports the health and wellness of our bodies, which mirror back gentle, loving calm.

The more complete Reiki principles, the Gainen, also suggest healthier ways to live our lives. Perhaps what makes the Gainen even more compelling as guidelines for daily life is that Mikao Usui gave them two titles—one that promises happiness, the other health. Here is a translation of the Gainen:

THE SECRET METHOD OF INVITING HAPPINESS

The Miraculous Medicine for All Diseases

> *Just for today, do not anger.*
> *Just for today, do not worry.*
> *Be grateful.*
> *Do your best.*
> *Be kind.*

*Morning and evening, with hands in gassho (prayer position)
and mind in focus, recite these principles for improvement of
body and mind.*

MIKAO USUI, FOUNDER
USUI REIKI RYOHO

The principles encourage us to choose peace when we are confronted with challenge or difficulty; to choose serenity when worldly concerns tempt us to feel overwhelmed; to appreciate each moment of our lives; to be guided by our own highest wisdom; and to be compassionate to all. Even in their more complete form, the Reiki principles are not commandments, but gentle suggestions. If we remind ourselves of them morning and night, if we remember them throughout the day, if we use Reiki when we are cast into emotional and mental turmoil by some unforeseen event, we can recover emotional well-being and mental calm— we can enjoy the precious gifts of happiness and peace of mind.

SUPPORTING A CLIENT'S MENTAL AND EMOTIONAL HEALING

When you work with a Reiki client, share the experience of the energy with a smile, with a kind word, with the gentleness of your touch. And assist the client in progressing toward recovery by being clear that you are here to serve by doing Reiki. Listen to your hands. Allow them to remain in position for as long as the client's body calls for the energy. In this way, the flow of the energy into the client can calm his heart, and his heart can calm him on all levels of being, accelerating his healing and deepening his love of life.

If you recognize that your client has a lot of mental and emotional work to do in order to accept physical healing, it is usually best to allow him to come to this recognition on his own. This may mean that you treat your client regularly for months in companionable silence. When and if the client begins to recognize that he needs to review his way of thinking or acknowledge repressed feelings that have contributed to creating his illness, know your place as a treatment provider. Unless you are qualified through other certification or licensing programs, or through volunteer training in counseling, acknowledge that you can only counsel him as a friend might. If he says that he does regard you as a friend, you may listen to him and advise accordingly. Or you may instead be more comfortable indicating that you regard your relationship with him as a professional one, and you are prepared to refer him to therapists, support groups, or peer-group co-counseling so that he can obtain the kind of help he specifically needs and wants at this time. Do assure him that Reiki is already helping to create change in his mental and emotional state—or he would not be asking for such help.

At the start of each treatment session, you might say a prayer that the energy heal the client's mental and emotional states as well as his physical body, or affirm that complete and permanent healing occur on all levels of being. While the energy works in harmony with the innate intelligence of the universal life force within the client to bring healing wherever it is needed, your participation in the process can be more than the simple placement of your Reiki hands.

Although the client may regard the time required to do the mental and emotional work to support complete and permanent healing as long, assure him that it is of importance. As you continue to treat with hands-on Reiki (and perhaps learn and apply Reiki distant-healing techniques for mental and emotional healing), healing on all levels of being accelerates and recovery becomes a matter of time. The more frequently the client invites and accepts healing, the sooner the flow of energy is likely to be felt by him simply as love, as comfort, as touch that soothes the heart. This supports the client as he does the mental work through therapy or other methods of inner processing, quickening his progress in even this.

You might also invite the client to work on his own with meditation or bio-feedback, stress management techniques, affirmations, visualization, or prayer—whatever feels appropriate and comfortable to him. Be prepared to suggest books, teachers, or classes in your area that might help him to work on his own healing through these methods. In this way, the client can come to terms with himself as a spiritual being, and with his illness as an opportunity for life review and revision, making complete and permanent recovery much more likely.

A FEW WORDS ABOUT INTENTION

One day, in a hands-on Reiki class, a student, a practitioner, and I were treating another student with the hand positions for the back on the treatment table. In response to a question about intention, I asked them to try an experiment. I invited the practitioner who was assisting to try directing the flow of the energy, which was already strong through all our hands. I suggested that she picture, affirm, and pray, without revealing what she requested. A moment later, the student on the treatment table said, "Oh, I felt that! The energy just shot down from my shoulder blade to my hip and then to my sacrum." When asked what the practitioner had imaged and asked of the energy, she said, "I pictured the energy as a stream of cobalt blue triangles that moved like a pool ball shot straight from her shoulder blade to her hip, and then to her sacrum." This was certainly clear validation that we could apply intention in a number of ways to working with the Reiki energy, with some success. However, when the practitioner stopped visualizing, affirming, and praying—that is, consciously intending—the energy continued to flow through her hands, resuming the steady, strong coursing that had preceded our experiment.

This was a good demonstration of how a Reiki practitioner can work with creative expressions of intention in cooperation with the energy. At the same time, it underlined the simple truth that the practitioner's intention does not matter. Given an opportunity to create healing, the energy will heal, whether the practitioner works with a conscious intention or not.*

Traditional Reiki masters teach, as Takata taught, that the practitioner's intention does not matter. Beyond applying the hands to the area in need of treatment, there is nothing the practitioner needs to do in terms of centering, grounding, calming, or controlling the mind. The energy will make all the adjustments necessary within the practitioner to create healing. Helen Haberly writes in *Reiki: Hawayo Takata's Story*: "Mrs. Takata emphasized it is simple, it is natural, it is scientific. There is no magic involved, no 'hocus pocus,' nor is there a need to create an altered state of consciousness in order to do this work. It is well to remain focused on the treatment, but Reiki will work automatically whenever the hands are applied to the area of need."[11]

Understanding and accepting this concept has permitted me (and many

---

*Helen Haberly who was a student and close friend of Takata's, conveys her teacher's convictions emphatically: "The practitioner has no control over what will happen, as the responsibility for whatever occurs lies with the one being treated. . . . The practitioner does not create this energy, but is simply the channel through which it is transferred; and in accepting this role of vessel, there is no attachment to results. One does not become a healer, for Reiki is the healer."[10]

others) to do Reiki in the midst of chaos and trauma, as well as when I am "of two minds"—focusing consciously on a conversation when I am giving a hands-on treatment, or on a book or a movie, while my hands flow with the energy to send distant healing. I have done so without guilt over this lack of focus, because I understand that neither I ("the ego" or personality with which I identity) nor my conscious mind, which carries thoughts of health and illness, and much else besides, does the work of healing. The Reiki energy works through me, despite my lack of focus and changing moods, as Spirit guides—with an intelligence much greater than my own and compassion beyond my comprehension.

How? What I understand from years of practicing Reiki—which have only reinforced the traditional Reiki master's instruction that the practitioner's intention does not matter—is that the four attunements required to practice hands-on Reiki healing establish a safe, stable conduit for healing energy below the threshold of the conscious mind. It is for this reason that practitioners sometimes report their hands turning on spontaneously while they sleep, or when they walk into a crowded room, or when they sit at their workshop table whittling or sewing. It is also for this reason that the practitioner's attention may wander as he does a client treatment without any change in the flow of the energy, except those dictated by the client's need. And it is for this reason that the practitioner, as well as the client, can gradually heal on all levels of being.

Because my mind is one that often wants scientific explanations, I have wondered whether the four attunements that establish the Reiki healing channel are much like programming a computer; perhaps repetition "conditions" the energetic pathways, just as it does the route an electrical impulse travels across the tiniest silicon chip. What does seem clear is that Reiki is "set" into the practitioner as deeply as the heart rate, respiration, blood pressure—all of which also usually work below the level of conscious intention, through the autonomic nervous system. (While we can develop the ability to regulate our breathing or steady our heartbeat or lower our blood pressure, we can't stop these functions through our intention—nor can we stop the flow of Reiki.)

This gives us an axis of intention that is understandable in terms of involuntary and voluntary functions. For a traditionally trained practitioner, the flow of Reiki is involuntary. We can, however, have some mild influence, just as with the involuntary functions of our body: with breathing, we can deliberately slow or speed up or hold the breath. With Reiki we can allow ourselves to come into harmony with the flow through our hands, and we can, with our conscious mind, visualize, affirm, or pray for a certain healing effect.

This means that the mental work of healing necessary for a complete and permanent recovery can be accomplished much more easily for the practitioner, because of the fundamental change created at the innermost level of being—an open heart and a reawakened connection to the source of life. Using Reiki to work with the mind and body becomes simple:

To change your life, change your mind.

To change your mind, change your heart.

To change your heart, use Reiki, and allow the energy of unconditional love to flow through you and transform you. When you think of it, add the power of prayer; when you think of it, work with visualization and affirmation. Always, continue to use Reiki and enjoy the self-healing that gradually, but inevitably, does come.

REIKI AND THE WILL OF THE SOUL

Reiki will not interfere with the will of the soul, although in time it transforms even the resistant heart and mind, bringing a sense of emotional and spiritual recovery to many who begin treatment while they are in their last days of life. Should this be the case, Reiki will bring relief from severe pain and a sense of peace and acceptance. Sometimes the practitioner, as well as the client, must learn and accept that death is also, in its way, healing. The final lesson of the mind and body is one of return to the same loving universal life force that birthed us and that sustains us each day of our lives. With the comprehension of that lesson comes awareness of new possibilities that we may glimpse through the stories of near-death survivors, who describe a feeling of overwhelming love and hope, and those who remember previous reincarnations and can provide details of their former day-to-day lives. As we learn more about who and what we are, and we begin to know ourselves as souls and energetic beings as well as individuals with physical bodies, names, addresses, families, and jobs, we may come to look upon death as a time for celebration. Coming around to that way of thinking may just be a matter of changing our minds.

8

PRACTICAL HUMAN
ANATOMY

DEEPENING AWARENESS, AWAKENING SENSITIVITY

The third attunement, which is done in the same way as the first and second, invites the students to a deeper awareness of the Reiki energy, sometimes through an experience that is uniquely individual, sometimes through an experience that is shared. Students sitting beside each other sometimes report hearing the same sound, such as a temple gong, or seeing the same view, as if they sat beside each other not only in the Reiki classroom but also in other dimensions of space and time.

> *"I felt you moving around me. I could feel something like a cone of light that came down over my head when you were standing behind me. I can still feel it. I can feel my hands, too. They feel kind of sparkly."*
>
> *"That's a good word for it. Sparkly hands. Like I was moving them over a glass of ginger ale. And warm all over. I'm going to have to take off this jacket."*

"Peaceful. I feel warmth all the way from my hands up to my shoulders."

"I was thinking about my daughter. She's away at college right now, but I kept thinking that she would really like this class. She would like being able to do this. My hands feel about the same as they did the last time—warm all over."

"I don't know if I feel different than the last time. But I feel really relaxed and good. My hands feel full of energy. Why don't they teach this in high schools?"

"That felt quieter than the first and second attunements. I do feel a lot more energy in my hands, though."

As the students realize that their awareness of the flow of Reiki energy through their hands is deepening and their perceptions of subtle sensations are growing keener, they begin listening on multiple levels: they listen very attentively to their hands and, in a more relaxed way, to the Reiki master. This is an appropriate time for the teacher to briefly review human anatomy. Although no one needs to know anatomy to use Reiki, some knowledge of how the body works and what its parts are called can be quite useful. There are three good reasons to gain this basic understanding: to cope with referential pain; to describe your experience clearly to conventional medical practitioners; and to understand the intuitive impressions you may receive about the nature of a client's medical condition.

Referential pain is pain that occurs at a distance from the site of injury or infection. For instance, many of the more than two hundred varieties of the herpes virus create referential pain. Once contracted, the virus lives dormant in the nerves at the place where the nerves exit the vertebrae of the spine. When a person who has contracted the virus becomes tired or stressed, the virus will move out along the nerve to a remote site and cause lesions, blisters, or redness and rash. Reiki hands can lessen the pain of shingles, which is caused by a herpes virus, by being applied over such inflammation, but they are much more effective in speeding healing if applied directly over those vertebrae of the spine that cover the roots of the infected nerves.

Referential pain can sometimes deceive the practitioner into thinking that he has treated the cause of a medical condition, when all he has done is alleviate the symptoms to a small degree. While the origin of most pain may be obvious, it is worth keeping in mind that both infection (such as herpes) and injury (such as carpal tunnel syndrome) can cause referential pain. If you are in doubt that Reiki healing is occurring as quickly as you would expect on the basis of past treatment experience, go to your local library and look in *The Merck Manual* to read about the condition you are treating. When you return to do additional treatments, adjust your hand placement, if necessary, to treat not only the symptomatic effects of the infection or injury, but the cause. You are likely to make much more rapid progress.

Because Reiki often does make progress in treating people who have not had success with allopathic medicine, it makes sense for Reiki practitioners to open a dialogue with an attending physician or nurse if that person seems receptive. The results of Reiki work on patients in hospitals and hospices speak for themselves, and research studies are ongoing through the National Institute of Health's Office of Alternative Medicine, but some physicians and nurses are still unaware of Reiki. For this reason, being able to speak knowledgeably and from practical experience can be of considerable value to all concerned.

Many Reiki practitioners also find that after their hands-on training, they begin to "see" flashes of what is going on inside the body in an intuitive way. For example, a practitioner might receive an impression of a change in the diameter of the intestines as she works on a client's abdomen. If she knows that, indeed, the intestines do change in diameter as they progress from the stomach to the colon, she can move on to understanding other details of the image she sees without feeling disconcerted by something quite normal. Such impressions can be more comfortably received when the practitioner has a knowledge base with which to make sense of them.

For all these reasons, learning basic human anatomy and becoming comfortable with the terminology used to describe the parts of the body is worthwhile. Not only can developing this knowledge base make you more effective as a practitioner, but it can also enable you to communicate more clearly to your client, and to any attending medical personnel also involved in your client's care. With confidence in your ability to present your experience in an articulate manner and your experiential knowledge of the healing work accomplished by the Reiki energy, you will project a professionalism as an alternative health care practitioner that your clients and your colleagues will find worthwhile.

126

BASIC I, THE FRONT OF THE TORSO

Basic I covers the front of the body, specifically the skin, muscles, bones, and organs located between the slight rise of bone called the xiphoid process at the base of the sternum, and the top of the pubic bone. Within this area are the viscera—the organs of digestion, metabolism, and excretion, the internal organs of reproduction, the hormone-secreting adrenals and pancreas, and the blood-purifying and antibody-producing spleen (see figure 8.1 on page 128). Stomach, liver, pancreas, gall bladder, intestines, kidneys, and ureters work together to digest, store, and distribute nutrients and dispose of waste products. Most perform essential roles, although there is some "system redundancy." For instance, kidney function can be maintained when only two-thirds of one kidney works.

These organs serve each other, as well as the whole body, in complex harmony. For example, when the stomach empties food into the small intestine, accompanying stomach acid stimulates the intestinal wall to produce a chemical messenger (called secretin), which is carried in the bloodstream to the pancreas. The pancreas responds by releasing acid-neutralizing pancreatic juice into the intestine, which triggers the further breakdown of the food into more usable form. Then the intestines send the nutrient-rich blood to the liver, which acts like a warehouse and shipping center for the body's fuel supply (and serves many other roles as well).

Supporting these many bodily functions, the aorta and the vena cava (the major blood vessels paralleling the spine) and their branches circulate blood; nerves relay information; and the pancreas and adrenal glands secrete hormones to target organs, tissues, and cells to sustain ongoing activities and to trigger emergency readiness.

Basic I upper-body "extras" include the heart, lungs, breasts, and the infection-fighting thymus gland, located behind the breastbone. Basic I lower-body "extras" include the middle of the abdomen over the reproductive organs, and the "hinges" where the torso joins the thighs. In this area, the femoral arteries and veins circulate blood to and from the legs, and many lymph glands manufacture antibodies and destroy and disperse the residues of infection.

Reiki can be of great value in maintaining or restoring the normal, healthy function of these organs and tissues because it works in harmony with the innate intelligence of the body, revitalizing the cells with universal life-force energy and recalling the presence of health.

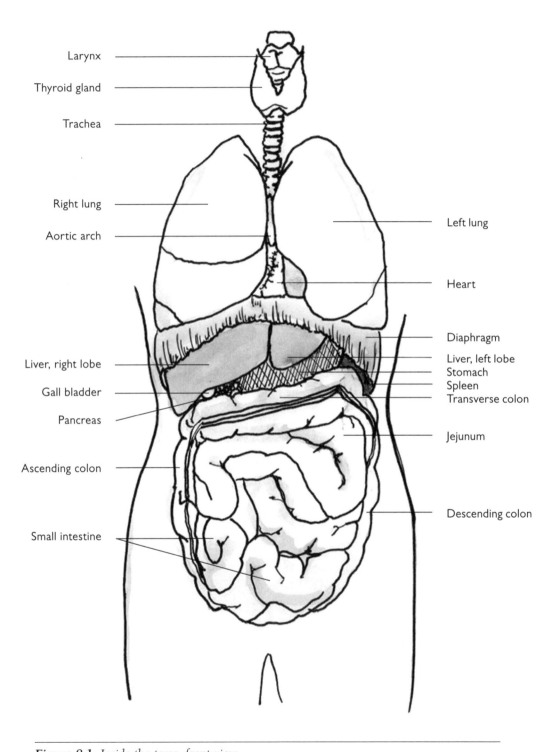

Larynx

Thyroid gland

Trachea

Right lung

Aortic arch

Left lung

Heart

Diaphragm

Liver, right lobe

Liver, left lobe
Stomach
Spleen
Transverse colon

Gall bladder

Pancreas

Jejunum

Ascending colon

Descending colon

Small intestine

Figure 8.1. *Inside the torso, front view*

BASIC II, THE HEAD

Basic II covers the head in four standard positions, from first position over the forehead and eyes to fourth position at the back of the skull. Within this area are the brain and the primary sensory organs: the eyes, the ears, the nose, and parts of the mouth and skin, all with nerve pathways connecting them directly to the brain for rapid processing of sensory information. Also within this area is the bulbous end of the spinal cord, called the brain stem, which supports involuntary and essential life functions such as heart rate and respiration. The brain's intense level of activity is maintained by a strong flow of glucose and oxygen-rich blood circulating through the large carotid arteries and jugular veins (on the sides of the neck) and many smaller arteries and veins as well.

The brain is the task-master organ, and in the interest of survival of the species, it is carefully housed. Cushioning and protecting the brain from blows from the front, from above, from the sides, and from the back are all the bones

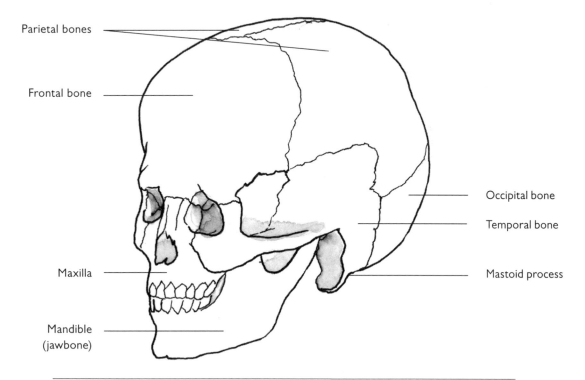

Figure 8.2. *The bones of the skull*

of the skull: the frontal, parietal, temporal, and occipital bones (see figure 8.2). The leathery membrane called the dura, and the cerebrospinal fluid, which flows through the dura, provide a soft cushion around the brain. Finally, guarding the brain from blows from below is the bony, segmented, spinal column, which acts like a shock absorber to moderate and disperse the force of physical impact through flexion, extension, and alignment of the vertebrae and disks.

The most recently evolved and largest part of the brain (protected by the frontal, parietal, and temporal bones of the skull) is the cerebrum or the "gray matter," the seat of conscious thought, voluntary actions, sensory awareness, and deliberate movement (see figures 8.3 and 8.4). The cerebrum is divided into left and right hemispheres; the hemispheres are joined by many fibrous bands containing nerve bundles, the neural pathways that communicate information between the hemispheres.

While the gray matter of both hemispheres looks much the same, there is little overlap of functions. The acts of speaking, reading, and writing are usually governed by the left hemisphere; musical and artistic abilities and

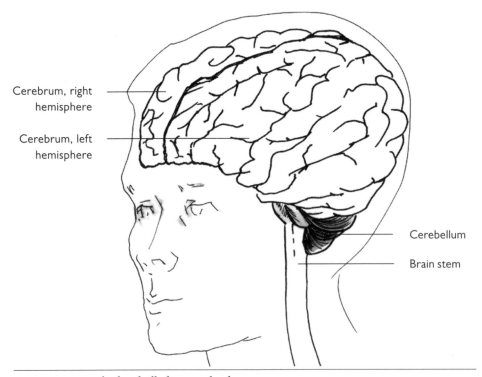

Figure 8.3. *Inside the skull, front and side view*

creative thought most often originate in the right hemisphere. Awareness of sensations on the right side of the body is usually registered in the left hemisphere, and vice versa; deliberate movement on the right side of the body is governed by the left hemisphere, and vice versa.

Covered by the occipital bone at the back of the skull, the cerebellum or "little brain" is a much older part of the brain in the evolutionary time line. This part of the brain is known to govern coordination and smooth-muscle movements. The cerebellum extends out of the back of the brain stem (see figure 8.5); both cerebellum and brain stem are joined to the bottom of the cerebrum by a fibrous band of connective tissue housing more neural pathways. Together these form the hindbrain, which supports involuntary and essential functions such as heart rate, respiration, and circulation, as well as balance at rest and in motion.

In the midbrain area is a tiny but powerful pea-shaped gland called the pituitary gland. Above and behind the pituitary, the hypothalamus sorts out

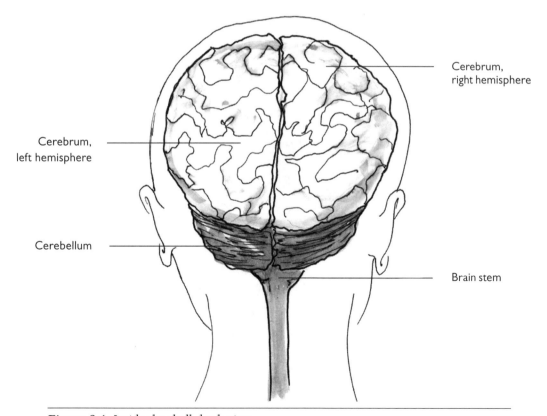

Figure 8.4. Inside the skull, back view

131

the complex sets of messages sent by the nervous and endocrine systems, and the thalamus routes information from the sense organs. Recent research using brain-scan technology shows that memory, long thought to be a "higher thinking" function occurring in the cerebrum, actually activates the midbrain.[1] In the very back of this protected space, the pineal gland serves its function. Mysterious to Western medical practice, this gland is linked to the opening of the "third eye" and intuitive awareness by those who practice meditation in the Eastern tradition.

While this description of the functions of the various parts of the brain is, at most, quite basic, it hints at the vast complexity of this organ and its relationship to every essential and nonessential "life-support" system in the body. (The regularity of the heartbeat is essential; the neural path a logical thought takes as it crosses someone's mind is not essential, but may contribute significantly to the quality of life.)

What is known about the brain is far exceeded by what is not known. In

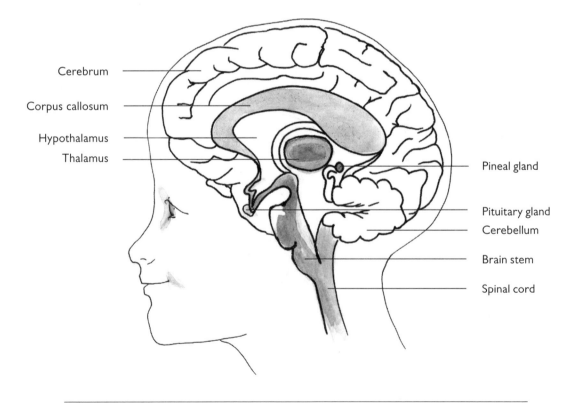

Figure 8.5. *Vertical cross-section of the brain*

this regard as well, Reiki-attuned hands may be of help not only to practitioners but also to medical researchers. Reiki hands recognize that the cerebellum may have a role to play in immune-system functions that scientists have not yet recognized. The extreme amount of energy drawn into the body in Basic II, position 4 when a client is HIV positive, or in other ways immune-system compromised, is an indication of this. (Could the same mechanisms that primitive man used to successfully ward off ancient forms of viral, bacterial, and fungal infections be located in the cerebellum? Could those mechanisms be activated by exposure to modern equivalents of these organisms? Or, at an even deeper level of the brain, could the hypothalamus be mediating these thoughts and feelings that are concerned with survival? By raising such questions Reiki extends the possibilities for research, as well as the pragmatic limits of healing.)

Like Basic I, the four positions of Basic II direct Reiki energy to most, but not all, of the area of the body that the particular position treats; some of the area is treated indirectly, as the energy disperses itself. What is significant, however, is that Reiki energy, from any of the four positions of Basic II, can penetrate all the way into the midbrain, where the most subtle and essential system-regulators—the pituitary gland, the thalamus, the hypothalamus, and the pineal gland—are housed. For this reason, a complete Reiki treatment will usually include only four positions on the head. Of course, extra positions lower down on the head, on the face, and on the throat, can also be done to good effect.

BASIC III, THE BACK

On a client, Basic III covers the back of the body, from the thoracic vertebrae through the lumbar vertebrae to the sacrum and coccyx. When treated with the usual sequence of Reiki hand positions, a client in good health will have already received the benefit of the energy's flow directed into his body from the front; for this reason, the Basic III hand positions are usually completed the most quickly.

However, listening to your hands when treating the back is just as important as it is elsewhere: the long, wide bands of muscle that support the spine are as prone to knots of tension as muscles anywhere in the body— perhaps even more so, because they compensate for both the momentary jarring and the lasting traumas that the spine so often endures. The flexible spine, which allows us to move with so much freedom, consists of many small, hollow, interlocking bones called vertebrae; there are seven in the neck, twelve in the thoracic area, five in the lower back, another five (fused into a single bone) at the sacrum, and four (also fused) at the coccyx. These bones are our "bodyguards," bearing our weight and the brunt of every step we take, and also serving as protection for the spinal cord, the long mass of nerve fibers that is the body's message-relay system.

A severed spinal cord usually results in paralysis or death. Damage to the vertebrae or the intervertebral disks often causes extreme pain and reduced limb or organ function. Simple misalignment of the vertebrae causes pain of a less severe nature, but still sufficient to cause stress, which suppresses the immune system. The health of the back, the spine, and the spinal cord is essential to the health of the body.

Reiki can offer an excellent source of relief from back-muscle tension, which is often all that is necessary for a client to enjoy feeling good again. When more serious damage to the spine or spinal cord has occurred, Reiki can also offer hope. A commitment to daily or frequent Reiki treatments, a positive attitude, and patience can turn around a dire prognosis. If the client has the use of his hands, or when he regains them, he may increase his chance of complete recovery by learning Reiki and committing to daily self-treatment. Family members and friends should continue to assist the healing process in whatever ways they can, for someone with spinal damage literally needs to accept the support of others to heal. While the family structure may not initially provide such support, regrouping so that support can be comfortably offered and accepted can create a healing environment for everyone concerned.

Most practitioners find that as they begin to treat clients on a regular basis, their curiosity about the workings of the human body is aroused. They discover themselves turning first to articles about healing or human physiology in magazines, or wandering in the library stacks browsing through books on medical subjects. Even when practitioners do not make such conscious efforts to learn more about anatomy and physiology, the Reiki energy itself continues to gently educate them to the mystery of human life.

9

TREATING CLIENTS

Most people begin to treat family and friends on an informal basis before setting up even a part-time client practice. Unless you already have a massage or bodywork table, this usually means that you will "Band-Aid"—put your hands wherever it hurts—before you give anyone a complete Reiki treatment. When you do, you are likely to be sitting on a chair or a footstool while your friend lays face up and fully clothed on a living room couch; or you may stand while your friend stretches out, face up and fully clothed, on a dining room table (padded with blankets, please, both for hygiene and comfort); or you may sit beside or kneel on a bed beside your spouse who is stretched out in pajamas and ready for sleep.

While we must all begin from wherever we are in terms of Reiki practice, you will discover that you will quickly want to get a treatment table if you do not already have one. No footstool, no dining room chair, no bed is comfortable enough to allow you to do an hour and a half or two hours of Reiki without feeling some strain across shoulder and lower back muscles. Since your physical stress will draw from the energy that is flowing through you to the client, you will find that not only do you feel physical discomfort from poor posture, but you also will become less effective through the course of the treatment! For this reason, as soon as you can, you will probably want to invest in a sturdy, well-designed massage table, and take good care of it. More information on how to select a treatment table is included in chapter 10.

Even though your first client is likely to be someone who will not mind your inexperience and the informality of your treatment area, you can do a lot to put her mind at ease before the treatment begins. Besides simply describing that Reiki is a form of alternative healing that uses channeled energy and reassuring her that most people find it quite relaxing, letting your client know that she does not have to take off clothes may be a relief. Suggesting she loosen any tight clothing, remove constricting belts, shoes, and eyeglasses, and lay comfortably on her back with her arms at her sides is a good next step.

As you become more professional in your approach to your practice, you will discover that these same simple courtesies serve you and the client well. A way to extend that sense of courtesy even further is to provide the client with a brief explanation of what you will do during the treatment, and to let her know when you are actually about to physically touch her and begin the hand positions. Saying something like this will suffice: "I am going to be placing my hands on you in a series of standard positions starting just below your breastbone and covering your abdomen, then your head, and finally, after you have rolled over, your back. I will be keeping my hands in each position until I feel a change in the flow of the energy, a signal from your body that you have received what you need for now to do some healing. Then I will move to the next position and wait for the same change in the energy flow. While I do this, you may just relax. I can put on some background music, if you would like. You may talk or not, as you like. You may even want to just drift off to sleep; that's fine. Lots of people do.

"Please let me know if at any point I can do anything to make you more comfortable—if I can put a blanket or a pillow under your knees, for example. Let me know, too, if you would like to take a break to get a glass of water or to go to the bathroom. If you do, we'll just continue the treatment when you return."

By presenting your treatment plan to your client before you begin, you create a safe space in which to have discussion and foster healing. Given this kind of preview the client may feel freer to ask questions that would otherwise have gone unasked and created a minor level of tension; also, she may volunteer that this week while playing tennis she fell and hurt her left knee, or that bursitis in her shoulder has really been bothering her. This dialogue will enable you to attend to her needs for healing in a much more dedicated and efficient way. You will be able to provide her with a complete Reiki treatment, and, at her invitation, to take that healing into the territory that is normally untreated, but that, on this specific occasion, may be the source of her greatest symptomatic pain. Even though the intensity and direction of Reiki energy is not in your control, encouraging your client to participate in such treatment decisions supports her sense of being in charge of her own well-being. This sense of empowerment is important and can carry over into situations outside the treatment room, helping your client make healthy lifestyle changes.

Your gentle introduction to the Reiki treatment and encouragement to your client to express concerns and ask questions may create such a feeling of safety that the client becomes comfortable disclosing personal information or expressing emotions that need release. If this occurs, stay calm, for your steady hands and continuing gentleness will help the client to return to his own peaceful center. Continue the treatment, listen with compassion, and regard whatever is revealed as confidential.

Although your client may have made a formal appointment with you expressly for the purpose of receiving a Reiki treatment, at the moment that you actually begin, ask for permission to touch. Reiki, like other forms of alternative healing and massage, occurs within the client's personal space. Your client, however relaxed he appears, deserves to have this space respected and acknowledged. All you need to do as a practitioner is ask, "May I begin treatment now?"

WORKING ON A CLIENT

Once you have practiced the standard hand positions of Basic I, II, and III on yourself and have gotten used to "Band-Aiding" friends and family members, you will find it easy to give a complete Reiki treatment to a client. Basic I covers the same area on a client that it does on you: the front of the torso, from the lower rib cage through the abdomen to the tip of the pubic bone; Basic II covers the same areas of the head; Basic III covers the back. The only difference is that, because you can comfortably work on a client either from a standing or a seated position at a treatment table, the Basic III hand positions can start at the top of the shoulders and cover some upper body areas that are not reached from Basic I, including the heart and lungs. It is also natural to want to continue your treatment below the areas that can be reached from Basic I with hand positions covering the lower back. Usually seven hand positions will cover most adults' backs from the shoulders to the coccyx. It is good practice to include all seven in any full treatment; they are described here as Basic III, positions 1, 2, 3, and 4, and Continuing the Back, positions 5, 6, and 7.

Working on a client also offers the opportunity to do extra hand positions, if time allows. Although massage therapists and practitioners who work in clinical settings may want to limit the treatment to the standard hand positions only and the time for each position to two to three minutes (if working in a half-hour treatment slot) or five minutes (if working in a one-hour treatment slot), the best way to do a complete treatment will always be to listen to your hands, changing position only when you feel a shift in the flow of the energy to the area under them.

This means that a healthy, active client may indeed be treated in a half hour, but most people will require more time. An hour to an hour and a half for someone who has not received a treatment before is to be expected. As people return for additional treatments and are maintaining a higher level of health, you will be able to complete the treatment in a shorter period of time. Someone who requires an hour and a half to start may begin to need only an hour and twenty minutes or an hour and ten minutes; eventually, with regular (weekly or biweekly) treatments, that same person will probably be able to receive a complete treatment in forty or forty-five minutes. Just as in self-treatment, the length of client treatment time will depend on the initial state of wellness or illness, and will be modified as vitality increases and health is gradually restored.

If the client is willing to work with you in an open-ended way and leave the amount of time up to the wisdom of the Reiki energy and his own body, you have the opportunity to integrate extra hand positions that will be of specific benefit to the client into the complete treatment. Before you begin the treatment, ask about the client's time constraints and whether there are any particular areas of the body that he would like to have treated. Generally, extra positions on the front torso or front extremities are done after Basic I; extra positions on the neck, throat, and head are done after Basic II; and extra positions on the back of the body are done after Basic III. For this reason, descriptions of the extra hand positions that may be done at each station of the treatment table are presented immediately following the required standard hand positions for Basic I, Basic II, and Basic III.

THE FRONT TORSO—BASIC POSITIONS

Basic I, Position 1 (Figure 9.1)

You might say, "To start the treatment I am going to locate your xiphoid process, which is a little raised mound of bone at the bottom of the breastbone, just above the diaphragm." If the client seems at all uncertain, take her hand and place it over your own xiphoid process, which she will be able to feel through your clothes. Once she is reassured, let her know you are going to start the treatment by saying, "I am going to begin now." Then gently feel with your fingertips for the base of the breastbone and the xiphoid process. (Remember that it may be either knobby or flat.)

Once you have located this point, imagine a horizontal line that extends across the body, and let this define the top of the Basic I treatment area. Lightly place your hands just below this line, over the diaphragm and the lower rib cage. It does not matter which of your hands is closest to you and which is furthest away. The fingertips of the hand close to you should just touch the base of the palm of the hand that is further away. Keep the fingers of both hands together, thumbs against palms. When you place your hands correctly on the

Figure 9.1

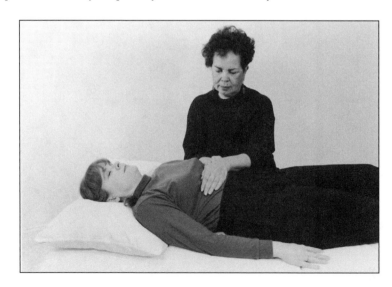

client in this position, you will find you can quite comfortably send Reiki.

You will be sending healing energy to skin, muscles, and bones of the lower rib cage; the organs of the lungs, liver, and stomach; and more deeply to the pancreas and spleen; and deeper still, to adrenal glands and kidneys, abdominal aorta and vena cava, and the nerve pathways that transit this area of the body from the spinal cord. Your client is likely to simply relax beneath your hands as the Reiki energy flows here. If the client is under a lot of stress, expect to spend a fair amount of time in this position before you feel a decrease in the flow, signaling that it is time to move on.

Basic I, Position 2 (Figure 9.2)

Moving through the positions of Basic I (and for that matter, of Basic II and III as well) is considerably easier to do on a client than it is on yourself. When you treat a client, you are likely to be standing or sitting comfortably, so that you are able to lay your hands on the client in Basic I, position 1 without straining at the shoulders or twisting at the waist. Still, if the client's need for healing is such that you must maintain this position for twenty minutes or even longer, you may discover that your upper arms are tiring, and your shoulders are tensing from the effort. The movement to Basic 1, position 2 should relieve these effects.

When you feel the decrease in the energy flow through your hands in Basic I, position 1, simply slide the hand that is furthest away from you across the client's abdomen toward you (like the top to bottom diagonal of the letter X) so

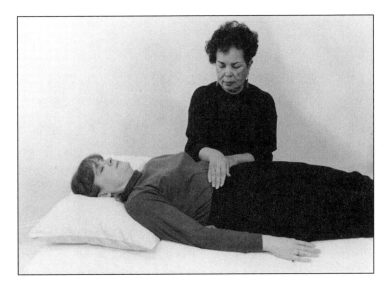

Figure 9.2

that it is side by side with the hand closest to you; then move the hand closest to you up across the client's abdomen (like the bottom to top diagonal of the letter X) so that your hands again span the client's body in a long line. It does not matter which of your hands is near to you and which is furthest away. As before, keep the fingers of both hands together and thumbs against palms.

When you place your hands correctly on the client in this position, you will be sending Reiki energy to the lower part of the stomach and the liver; to the pancreas, gall bladder, and upper intestines; to the kidneys and ureters; and to the major arteries, veins, and nerve pathways that support these organs. Many clients enjoy the relaxing effects of being treated with Reiki energy in this position. If their appointment for treatment follows lunch or dinner, however, they may be surprised at the gurgling noises the stomach makes under your hands. Simply assure them that they are enjoying the acceleration of a natural process—digestion—and move your hands when the change in the energy signals you to do so.

Basic I, Position 3 (Figure 9.3)

Moving from Basic 1, position 2 to Basic I, position 3 is accomplished with as much ease as the last position change. Again, follow the X pattern, only this time move the hand closest to you up across the client's abdomen first so that it comes to rest, for a moment, beside the hand that was furthest from you in the second position. Then, maintaining light contact, slide the hand that was

Figure 9.3

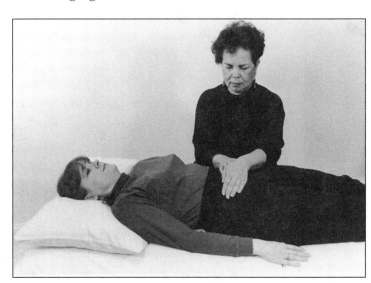

farthest from you in the second position down across the client's abdomen so that it comes to rest beneath the other hand, close to you. Both hands will now be in the same positions relative to each other that they were in Basic I, position 1. However, they will be resting over a different area of the abdomen—the midsection of the body, roughly over the navel and the waistline—the same area that your hands rest when you treat yourself in Basic I, position 3.

This is both the "belly laugh" and the "bellyache" position. (My teacher said Takata termed this area "the emotional radio.") Hands-on here can relax and relieve emotional stress, so often expressed in physical symptoms such as nausea or indigestion. Directed Reiki here can also bring up energy blockages for release, usually perceived by the client in the form of a passing sensation of pain, rather like a stitch in the side from running hard and becoming winded. Feeling any sensation of pain during a Reiki treatment is so rare that it is usually quite startling and alarming to the client. Simply explain to the client what is occurring and assure him that the pain will pass within a minute or two. It always does.

The client will receive the healing effects of the Reiki energy directly into the small intestines, the ascending and the descending colon, the ureters, the inferior mesenteric artery, the inferior vena cava, lesser arteries and veins, and many nerve pathways. The client may also experience sensations of Reiki energy radiating out from this position to other parts of the body.

Basic I, Position 4 (Figure 9.4)

If your client is not a standard four-position size, simply do additional paired hand positions until you reach this area of the abdomen, then move your hands into a wide-angled V, joining them, if the client is female, fingertips to palm, just above the client's pubic bone. If the client is male, move you're hands into a wide-angled V, a few inches above the physical body to maintain safe and appropriate boundaries. Depending upon how you placed your hands to begin the treatment, you may be able to simply slide your hands down from position 3 into position 4, or you may have to switch their relative positions before moving into position 4. In either case, your hands should come to rest comfortably just inside the client's pelvic cradle.

This is the area of the body in which the processes of digestion, elimination, and reproduction all occur. The intestines, the colon, the ureters, and the urinary

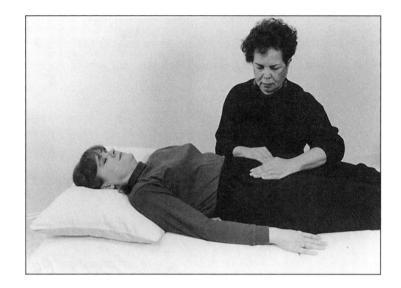

Figure 9.4

bladder receive direct benefit. Women also absorb healing into the uterus, cervix, vagina, fallopian tubes, and ovaries; men experience healing effects to the prostate gland, seminal vesicles, and the vas deferens. Deep under these organs, the client's sigmoid colon and rectum may also draw Reiki energy.

OPTIONAL POSITIONS

If time allows and the client has agreed to take advantage of the opportunity, using a few well-chosen extra hand positions can do a lot to increase the client's satisfaction with the treatment. For example, a client who knows that he has a heart condition will probably feel slighted—and rightly so—if his heart is not directly sent a healing dose of Reiki energy, even if he has been assured that the energy disperses to wherever it is needed in the body. If a client has developed a medical problem in an area not directly treated by the standard hand positions, it is natural that symptom relief should be his first concern.

Some of the extra positions described below, such as the heart, are often requested. Some are not usually requested, but provide an important boost to the immune system or specific symptom relief. The hand positions described have been found to be comfortable for most practitioners as well as for clients. Some, such as the throat, are suggested with alternatives to allow for client preferences. (Many people dislike the sensation of having something touching the throat, and will not wear turtlenecks or sleep with the blankets touching this sensitive area.) Just as you can do the standard hand positions through layers of clothing, so you can also do any of these extra hand positions through layers of clothing, with no diminishment of the healing effects.

Heart (Figure 9.5)

After completing the four standard positions of Basic I, treat the heart with hands paired, side by side, over the breastbone and left chest. Keep fingers together, thumbs against palms. Attend to the flow of energy through your hands and wait until there is a clear downward shift in activity before moving to another position.

This position treats any heart condition, any circulation problem, and the referential pain (via the vagus nerve to the stomach) of heartburn and indigestion. Systemic infections that are blood-borne, and some autoimmune conditions, such as allergies, also benefit greatly from treatment of the heart.

Thymus T (Figure 9.6)

Place one hand horizontally across the notch of the client's collarbone and the other hand perpendicular to the first over the breastbone (sternum) to treat the thymus gland, which is involved in fighting infections and disease conditions of all kinds.

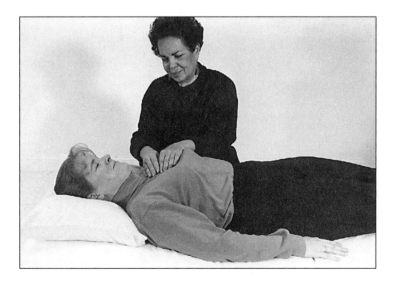

Figure 9.5

Breasts (Figure 9.7)

If the client has specifically requested treatment of the breasts (which often happens when a problematic mammogram or biopsy has occurred), discuss in advance whether or not hands-on healing feels safe and appropriate; consider whether you, as a practitioner, feel comfortable with hands-on healing in this area. If not, work in the energy field, at least a couple inches above the breasts to maintain the client's sense of safety, as well as your own sense of appropriate boundaries and professionalism.

The breasts are most easily treated as an extra position; do them as an extra position after completing Basic I standard positions. Because this is a more intimate area than others treated, and because some of the clients who come to you may have suffered sexual abuse, do rouse or wake your client to let her know that you are about to touch her breasts, and do so in as non-threatening a manner as you are able. Use a gentle but firm touch, keeping your fingers together and thumbs against palms as for any Reiki position on a client. Treat each breast individually, using two or three hand positions to complete the circle. There is no need to treat the nipple unless the client has specifically requested that you do so.

Should your hands indicate any unusual variation in the Reiki energy flow to the breast tissue, urge your client to see a doctor for a mammogram. If the client is requesting treatment of her breasts because she has been diagnosed with fibrocystic

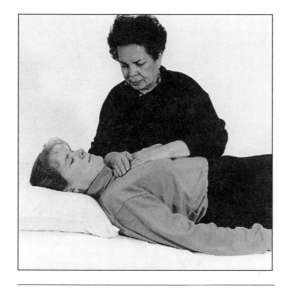

Figure 9.6

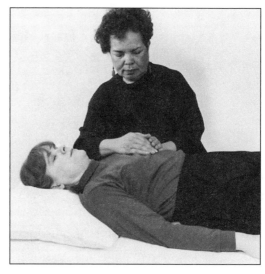

Figure 9.7

breasts, urge her to follow her doctor's recommendations regarding dietary changes and follow-up care. If the client has recently had a biopsy, been diagnosed with a benign or malignant tumor, or has undergone breast cancer surgery or radiation treatment, ask if she would like you to work in the energy field above the breast rather than directly on it. If you allow your hands to float an inch or so over the affected area, the Reiki energy will flow just the same, with just as much healing effect, and your client may be more comfortable during the process.

The client may tell you that she feels pain in the area of the biopsy or surgical incision, or that her skin itches; these are natural responses both to the course of healing and to the stimulus of the Reiki energy. Severed or damaged nerves charged to some further work of healing may convey an initial message to the brain of discomfort. Urge your client to bear the momentary sensation, if possible, as it will shortly change.

A client who comes for Reiki treatment who has endured life-threatening illness often needs to reflect on her lifestyle and make healthy changes. Since complete and permanent healing can only occur if the cause or causes of a medical condition are acknowledged and understood, support her work on herself with attentive listening, unconditional acceptance of her as she is right now, and a positive attitude regarding her recovery. Reiki by itself sometimes works miracles, but you can assist the process by being fully present to your client, coming from your heart, and letting the light of your hands show her hope.

Upper Respiratory Tract (Figure 9.8)
Lay your hands in a long line across the client's upper chest area, so that the fingertips of the hand closest to you touch the base of the palm of the hand furthest away just under the notch or midpoint of the collarbone. When the area has received enough Reiki energy and the flow through your hands has diminished in intensity, do a second position (and a third on a person who is tall or has a large build) using the same X pattern of movements that you used to progress through Basic I, positions 1, 2, and 3.

These hand positions treat any acute respiratory tract infection, including chest colds, bronchitis, and pneumonia; they also ease the congested and constricted bronchial passages of allergy and asthma sufferers. While colds, bronchitis, and pneumonia may be regarded as acute, bronchitis and pneumo-

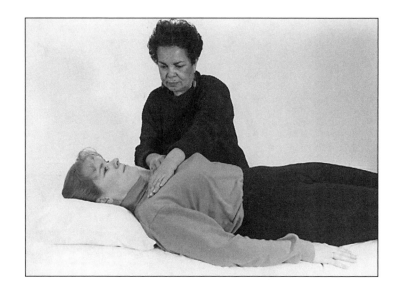

Figure 9.8

nia may become chronic without proper medical treatment. The client should be urged to work with his family physician and associated specialists to take advantage of the symptom relief that Western medicine can provide.

Allergies and asthma are chronic conditions, with episodic attacks in response to stress, cold, allergens (such as dust mites, mold, and pet hair), and chemical and environmental pollutants. A client who wants continued symptom relief from either of these conditions should learn to do hands-on Reiki himself and do self-treatment at least once a day, with focused attention on these areas.

Such conditions, which often take years to develop, can gradually improve with Reiki to the point where medications and bronchodilators are no longer needed on a regular basis. However, the progression of this improvement must be carefully monitored by a qualified medical doctor, and prescriptions gradually adjusted to reflect this improvement. Caution an allergic or asthmatic client who decides to learn Reiki that using intuition to decide that you no longer need prescribed medication or an inhalator is irresponsible and reckless self-endangerment and could prove fatal.

Shoulders (Figure 9.9)

Treat the shoulders one at a time, if the client requests they be treated, by simply wrapping your hands around the shoulder joint. On a child or a small woman, you may be able to cover the area in one position. On a larger woman

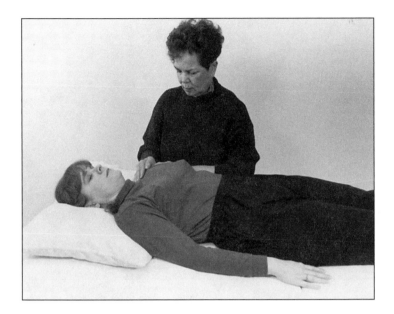

Figure 9.9

or on a man, you will need to move your hands to circle the joint completely.

Shoulder joints and muscles are definitely not all the same. Muscular shoulders may seem awkward to work around. Do your best. Well-developed, sore muscles appreciate Reiki energy just as much as less developed ones do. If your client works out at a gym and has adopted the philosophy of "no pain, no gain," you may draw the comment, "Oh, your hands feel like a heating pad." Consider this a compliment, and wait until the "heating pad" turns off before moving to another position.

Arms, Elbows, Wrists, Hands (Figures 9.10 and 9.11)

Clients may request that you work on a specific site of acute injury on the arms, elbows, wrists, or hands. Do so after completing Basic I and any other upper-body extras the client has requested you do (within the available time). It is easy to wrap both your hands around an injury site on the arms: simply put one hand over and one hand under the site. Use the same method to work on elbows or wrists that evidence joint pain. Use one hand under your client's hand and the other hand over your client's hand to comfortably work on hand injuries or muscle tension accumulated after a day at the keyboard or the workshop bench. With any of these extra positions, simply hold the position until you feel a decrease in the energy flow through your hands, and then move on.

148

If the client does not present an acute injury and yet has complained of symptomatic pain, remember that carpal tunnel syndrome (usually best treated on the wrists) causes referential pain to the fingers and the thumb, and all the way up the arm to the elbow and even to the shoulder. Carpal tunnel syndrome can be disabling, with ramifications that are far-reaching. Urge the client to see a doctor if he tells you that the pain has been present for some time. The doctor can prescribe an anti-inflammatory medication, if necessary, and a splint to keep the wrist immobilized.

A cut on a finger will need to be treated by holding the affected area with one hand. While you do this, do not waste your other hand. You might hold the client's wrist or even put your hand on your own midsection. The energy is flowing, so take full advantage of it. When the cut finger stops absorbing a significant amount of energy, move on and put both your hands back to work for the client.

Should the acute injury be a burn, remember that you can lift your hand above the affected area and the energy will flow with equal effectiveness. While the energy may not express itself as noticeable heat, if the client says the sensation is uncomfortable, this is a small accommodation to make to increase his comfort.

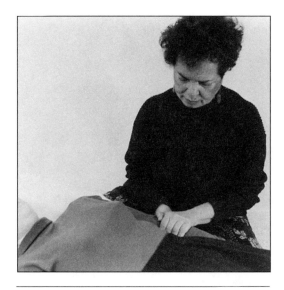

Figure 9.10

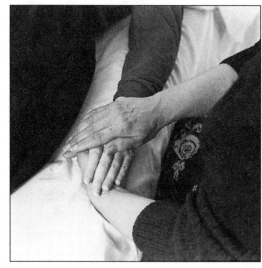

Figure 9.11

Abdomen (Figure 9.12)

If your client has requested some special attention to this area, after completing the V of Basic I, position 4, lay your hands, side by side, across the lower abdomen. This position is excellent for treatment of constipation, diarrhea, and the intestinal cramping that comes with stomach viruses.

Because it focuses healing energy directly to the reproductive organs, this position provides respite from menstrual cramps. It also enhances fertility in a woman who wishes to become pregnant, benefits a baby in utero, and helps to ease the intensity of labor in a woman giving birth. For many women, this is a favorite position.

"Hinges" (Figure 9.13)

This is an easy extra to do on a client immediately following completion of the standard four positions of Basic I. Simply widen the V used in fourth position to the point where each hand lays along the fold where the torso joins the leg. Should you be uncertain whether you are over the right area (which may happen with a client who is overweight), approximate the position with one hand and use the other to raise the client's leg slightly at the knee, giving the client a few words of advance notice that you will be doing so. Clothing will bunch into folds over the area, indicating the proper position for your hand. Once

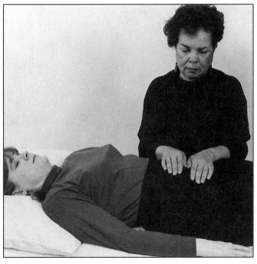

Figure 9.12   Figure 9.13

you have the first hand placed, remove your other hand from under the client's knee and move it to the same relative location on the other side of the client's abdomen to form your V.

This position offers help to those who have poor circulation in their legs or who have varicose veins. Because so many lymph nodes are situated here, there is also advantage in augmenting the standard positions with this one when you are treating a client who has been suffering from acute or chronic infection. As always, wait until you feel an entire cycle of the energy flow (hands turning on; increase in activity; stable, steady flow; decrease in activity) before moving to another position.

Legs, Knees, Ankles, Feet (Figures 9.14 and 9.15)

Occasionally clients request Reiki energy be sent to acute injury sites on the legs, but more usually the request is made to redress the imbalances of pulled muscles, torn tendons and ligaments, and sprained joints. Treatment of legs, knees, ankles, and feet is done along one side of the body at a time, in the same way you do the upper-body extremities: wrapping one hand over and one under, and using sufficient positions to circle the affected areas.

Knees benefit from placement of hands on the kneecap and on both sides of the kneecap, as well as over and under the joint. Ankles can usually

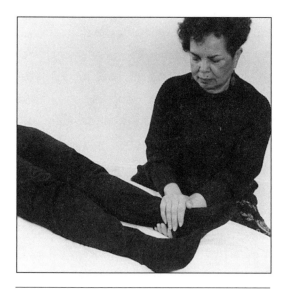

Figure 9.14

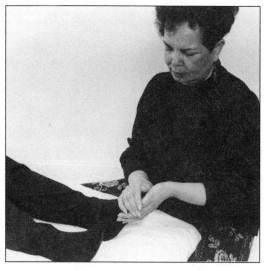

Figure 9.15

be comfortably circled in one hand position, one hand over and one under the joint. Feet are so often neglected that most people love the sensation of Reiki energy flowing into their toes, the balls of the feet, over and under the arch, under the heel, and behind the Achilles tendon. In treating feet from the front of the body, simply wrap your hands around the feet as comfortably as you can.

You may treat the client's lower body by working on one side and then the other, down to the feet, or you may work on one side, treat both feet at the same time, and then move to the other side. You may also decide to do the feet after doing Basic I, II, and III and all other extra positions. Because Reiki energy on the feet tends to draw the energy into the lower body and help the client to feel balanced and grounded as he returns to normal awareness, it is a wonderful way to end a treatment.

THE HEAD—BASIC POSITIONS

Basic II, Position 1 (Figure 9.16)

Basic II, position 1 on a client treats the same area of the body as you do in self-treatment of Basic II, position 1. Move from the side of the table to the head of the table; stand or sit, as you prefer. You should be directly behind the crown of the client's head.

If you have consistently listened to your hands throughout the treatment up to this point, your client may be deeply relaxed or even asleep, with eyes closed. To avoid startling him awake, softly say his name. When you have his acknowledgment, explain that you are going to begin to do the hand positions on the head. If your client has long hair, ask her to lift up her head from the pillow and gather her hair so that it flows back over the pillow and out of the way. Otherwise you will be continually concerned with trying not to pull the client's hair as you move from one position on the head to the next.

Once the client is comfortably situated on the pillow and is alert, let him know that you will be placing a folded tissue over his eyes so as not to tickle him. Follow up on this with unhurried action. Then gently place your hands down over the client's forehead and eyes, so that your thumbs touch over the client's forehead and your index fingers rest on either side of the client's nose.

The tips of your index fingers should be even with the base of his nose, but the client should be able to breathe easily.

You will find that this is a restful position to use for treating with Reiki, particularly if you are seated. You do not have to strain shoulders or back, and your wrists are supported by the pillow under the client's head. As with all the positions, listen to the energy in your hands through at least one complete cycle: wait until you feel your hands have turned on and are actively sending the energy; allow the energy to rise and stabilize at its own level of intensity; then wait for a downward shift in the intensity—your signal to move to the next position. Once you have completed this position you can remove the folded tissue from over your client's eyes.

This is the position of choice to treat headaches, sinus infections, eyestrain, allergy symptoms, and head colds, as well as serious diseases affecting the eyes, such as glaucoma or cataracts, and the frontal lobes of the brain, such as Alzheimer's disease. Depending upon the nature of the presenting symptoms, it may also be an active position for treatment of brain aneurysm and stroke. Anyone suffering from adult-onset epilepsy may draw heavily in the head positions, as may anyone who has an invasive tumor. (Sending Reiki energy to heal a tumor can be an odd experience. The blockage may not seem to draw at all initially; patience and perseverance are called for.) Diseases such as meningitis, which can infect the cerebrospinal fluid, may also create a strong sensation of

Figure 9.16

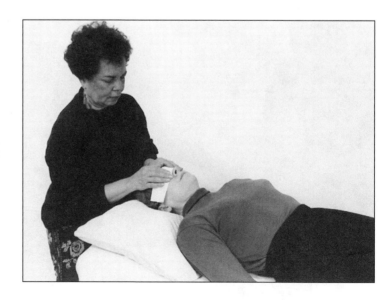

153

activity here, although the sensation is likely to be strongest nearer to the back of the head (and the brain stem and the spinal cord).

Basic II, Position 2 (Figure 9.17)

Going from Basic II, position 1 to Basic II, position 2 is easy. Allowing your little fingers to remain in contact with the client's head, raise your hands up and away from the client's forehead. Touch your thumbs to little fingers and allow your thumbs to assume the position occupied by the little fingers. Relax your hands and allow them to come to rest comfortably over the front and sides of the client's head, covering the temples.

This position is standard to continue a complete treatment. It is also of particular value in treating headache, sinus infections, eyestrain, neuralgia, allergies, head colds, and more serious conditions originating or presenting symptoms in the frontal and temporal lobes of the brain. As with all positions, allow your hands to send the healing energy until you feel the intensity of the energy flow clearly diminishing, and only then move to the next position.

Basic II, Position 3 (Figure 9.18)

Moving from Basic II, position 2 to Basic II, position 3 is accomplished with the same set of motions as for the last position. Using the little fingers of each

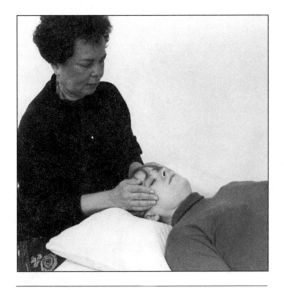

Figure 9.17

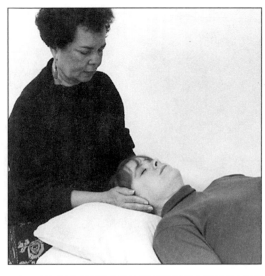

Figure 9.18

hand as a stable pivot point, swing your hands out, then touch your thumbs to little fingers and allow them to mark the place held by the little fingers. Relax your hands and allow them to come to rest lightly over the sides of the client's head, covering the ears.

This standard position is of help in treating ear infections, deafness, headache, sinus infections, allergies, head colds, neuralgia, and more serious conditions originating or presenting symptoms in the temporal and parietal lobes of the brain, or in the midbrain. For deeper level treatment, allow your hands to remain in position for more than one cycle of energy flow. For example, if you wish to treat earache accompanying a minor sore throat, attending the energy flow through one cycle is sufficient; if you wish to treat a hormonal imbalance originating in the pituitary gland, hold your hands in position through another cycle. While this is not absolutely necessary, it will create even more rapid healing of conditions originating at deeper levels.

Basic II, Position 4 (Figure 9.19)

Your client may have drifted away into dreams as you worked on his head to this point. Because the hand movements from position 3 to position 4 may be disruptive, you may want to rouse the client to let him know what you will be doing by saying his name. When you have a nod or murmur of acknowledgment, let the client know that you are going to be moving your hands under his head; he need not do anything at all except continue to relax.

Then move your hands, one at a time, from position 3, over the ears, to position 4, supporting the back of the head. To do this, simply use one hand to roll the client's head on the pillow, supporting it with the other. Then slide this hand down into the space that is opened up by the movement, so that your hand now cradles the client's head from just behind the ear to the midpoint at the back of the head. Then, using this hand for support, roll the client's head to the other side, slide your other hand down into the space opened by the movement, and then allow your client's head to come to rest in the hollows of both hands.

Although this may seem awkward at first, with practice it becomes quite easy. My teacher told us to imagine that we were rolling a melon in our hands. If the client is relaxed and not trying to help, this is indeed what these hand movements will feel like. If a client has long hair, be especially gentle as you

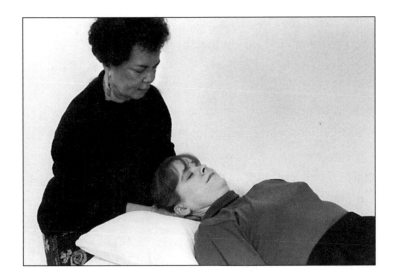

Figure 9.19

slide your hands into position. (If you helped the client gather her hair and pull it back over the pillow before starting the hand positions on the head, the length of her hair should not complicate matters.)

The fourth position is extremely important in treating anyone with infection of any kind, particularly those that compromise or suppress the immune system, such as HIV. (Although I can offer no documentation to bear this out, your properly attuned hands will give testimony to this effect.) Sinus and ear infections, colds, and cold sores (herpes simplex), and neuralgia also respond well to concentrated Reiki treatment here. This is a key position for treatment of meningitis, although it should be remembered that extra positions over the cervical vertebrae at the back of the neck and lower down over the spine and spinal cord will be of great benefit.

OPTIONAL POSITIONS

Jawbones and Teeth (Figure 9.20)

The lower sinuses, in the area under the eyes and the nose, are not as easy to do on a client as they are to do on yourself. While you can comfortably cover this area on yourself with your hands, adjusting the pressure of your touch so that you find it easy to breathe, doing the same on a client can be difficult.

For that reason, the lower sinuses are usually addressed with the same

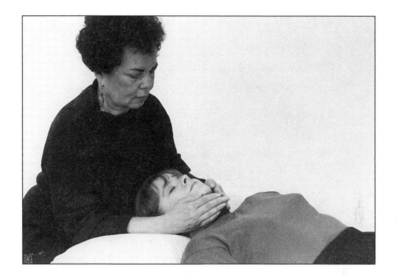

Figure 9.20

position used to treat the teeth and the jaw. Again, to do this position on a client, sit or kneel at the head of the treatment table. Allow your elbows to rest on the edge of the table and your forearms to relax on the pillow on either side of the client's head; place your hands along the client's jawline, so that your fingertips meet lightly under the client's chin. If a client specifically requests that you work directly on the lower sinuses, place a tissue over the mouth before resting your hands on either side of the client's nose. If this seems uncomfortable to you or the client, raise your hands up to an inch or so over the area, then let the energy flow.

Reiki here can provide symptom relief for those who have toothache, allergies, sinus or salivary gland infections, neuralgia, or ulcerative sores in or around the mouth or nose. If such sores are herpetic, make sure to treat the back of the head and the neck in order to address the infection at its source. In addition, so as not to spread infection, work in the energy field over the area rather than hands-on.

Front Throat and Thyroid (Figure 9.21)

To treat the client's throat and thyroid, sit or kneel at the head of the treatment table. Rest your elbows on the edge of the table and your forearms on the pillow on either side of the client's head; join your hands, at fingertips only, then simply allow the energy to flow through your hands into the surrounding area.

For clients who want special attention to the throat, comfortably support your forearms on the pillow on either side of the client's head, and then let your hands come together in a relaxed arch in the energy field over the throat. Most clients find the soothing relief the Reiki energy provides just as perceptible this way as with direct physical contact; and if the client is relaxed or dozing, working an inch or two above the throat is comforting and less intrusive than working hands-on.

This position sends Reiki energy to the skin, muscles, bones of the throat, salivary glands, lymph glands, and the thyroid and the parathyroid glands. It can provide gentle, rapid relief from sore throat, and direct targeted healing to more serious conditions, such as throat cancer and thyroid dysfunction.

Side Throat and Carotid Arteries (Figure 9.22)

Again, treating with Reiki in this position is best accomplished by the practitioner who is seated or kneeling at the head of the treatment table. With forearms supported on the pillow on either side of the client's head, place the hands on the sides of the neck, just under the ears. If this seems uncomfortable to the client, rest the backs of your hands on the pillow as well, so that the relaxed curve of your open palms and fingertips directs the energy to the lower part of the client's head, with focused flow to the sides of the neck, just under the ears.

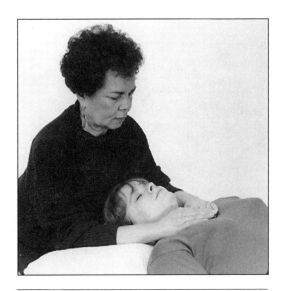

Figure 9.21

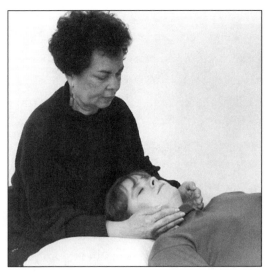

Figure 9.22

This is usually a very tension-relieving position, as the energy targets trigger-point pain in muscles and boosts circulation to and from the brain. When the client has had symptoms of any infection, treating with Reiki in this position will assist antibody production and lymph-node drainage from the many lymph nodes here. This is also an important position to use in treating anyone who has had a stroke or warning signs of a stroke. These include high blood pressure, heart disease, diabetes, and transient ischemic attacks, which are brief episodes of stroke symptoms—weakness, numbness, blurred vision, difficulty with speech (especially on one side of the mouth), unsteadiness, and/or severe headache.

Back of the Neck (Figure 9.23)

After receiving Reiki energy through all the standard positions of Basic I and II and a few extra positions, most clients on the treatment table will be deeply relaxed; some will be asleep. It is usually fairly easy for the practitioner to slip one or both hands under the client's neck, gently cradling the area while healing energy flows.

Although the back of the neck is certainly within the expected treatment area for Basic II, it may also be offered as an extra when the client is face down on the table, either before beginning treatment of the back or upon its completion. (One hand placed over the cervical spine and the other over the sacrum can help to bring about a sense of physical balance and alignment that many clients find very soothing.)

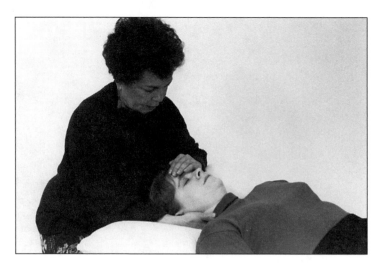

Figure 9.23

159

THE BACK—BASIC POSITIONS

Basic III, Position 1 (Figure 9.24)

By the time you have finished the standard and extra positions for Basic II, your client is likely to be lightly dozing. To treat your client in Basic III, you will need to move from the head to the side of the treatment table. This presents you with an opportunity to catch a quick stretch or a sip of water before going to your station.

To work on the back, you will need to have your client turn over. Again, this is likely to mean gently rousing him. After you have spoken his name, you might say something like this: "To continue the treatment, I need you to turn over. Please take your time. You can even keep your eyes closed, if you'd like, and just lean up, roll onto your side, and then gently lay down onto your stomach. You may want a pillow under your shins or under your chest so that the muscles in your back can relax more. May I get a pillow for you?"

After your client is comfortable again, you can begin doing the hand positions for Basic III. Rather than starting over the adrenal glands, take advantage of the opportunity to treat the often tense and sore muscles of the upper back. Do as many positions as necessary to cover the area from the trapezius muscles through the deltoids and the latissimus dorsi down to the gluteus maximus (see figure 9.25). On an adult client, this will usually mean approximately seven positions rather than four.

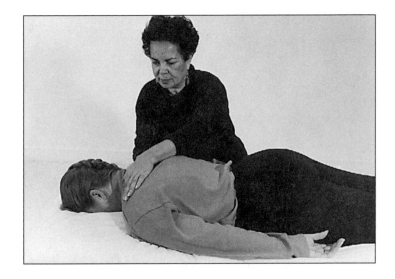

Figure 9.24

160

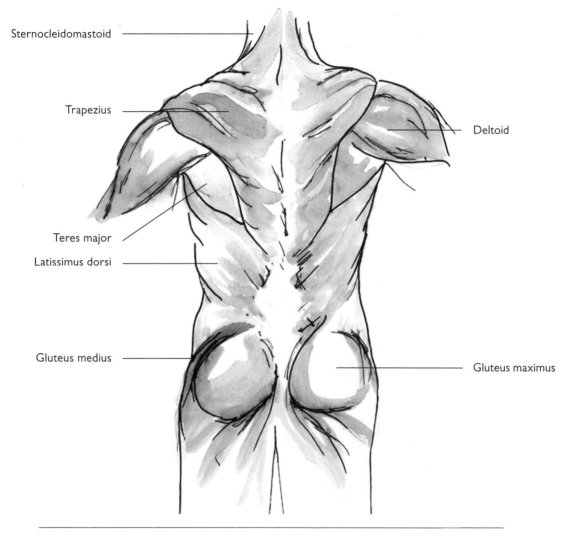

Sternocleidomastoid

Trapezius

Deltoid

Teres major

Latissimus dorsi

Gluteus medius

Gluteus maximus

Figure 9.25. *The muscles of the back*

To move into the first position, simply place your hands, end to end, in a line across the shoulders. Under your hands, the client's shoulder muscles should ease with the flow of the energy. (Many massage therapists trained in Reiki begin with their hands here to gently relax the muscles before manipulating them with more aggressive forms of bodywork, such as Swedish or deep muscle massage.) Upper respiratory passages, including the bronchi or the lungs, may open up if congestion has been present. The thymus gland may absorb healing energy as well.

Basic III, Position 2 (Figure 9.26)

Moving your hands into position 2 on the client's back is accomplished the same way as moving into position 2 on the front. Maintaining a light touch, simply glide the hand furthest away from you toward you, so that it comes to rest side by side the hand nearest to you in the first position. Then move that "anchor" hand further away, so that it forms a straight line (with the other hand) across the client's back.

You will be treating the broad span of the shoulder muscles (trapezius and deltoid) and the point where they come together (where knots of muscle tension often form). The rib cage, the aorta and vena cava, the heart, the pulmonary arteries and veins, and the lungs will receive direct benefit. This is an excellent position to use when circulatory or respiratory systems are in need of special healing, whether the condition is acute or chronic and the symptoms mild or severe.

Basic III, Position 3 (Figure 9.27)

Working your way through the positions on the client's back is like doing cross-stitch. Your hands keep moving in the X pattern that you first used on the front, doing Basic I. To equalize stress on your shoulders (whether you stand or sit to do the treatment), move the hand that is nearest to you up across the

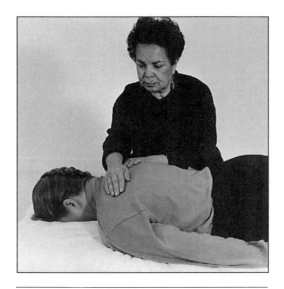

Figure 9.26

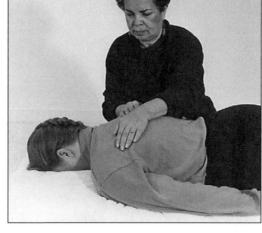

Figure 9.27

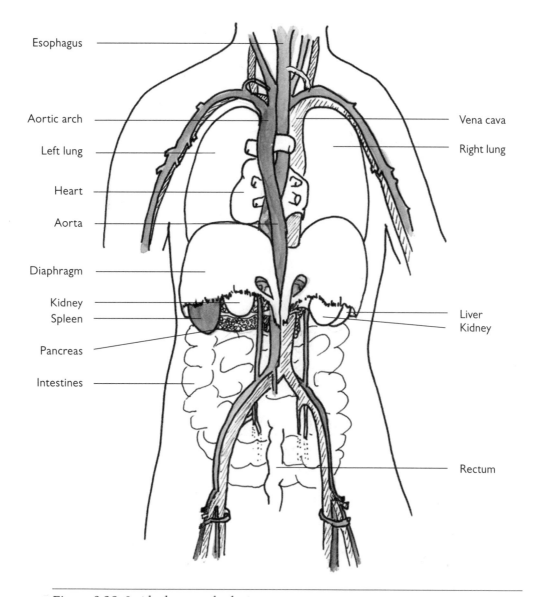

Esophagus

Aortic arch
Left lung
Heart
Aorta

Diaphragm

Kidney
Spleen

Pancreas

Intestines

Vena cava
Right lung

Liver
Kidney

Rectum

Figure 9.28. Inside the torso, back view

client's back so that it comes to rest side by side the hand furthest from you in the second position. Then move that hand toward you, so that it forms a straight line (with the other hand) across the client's back.

Here, the wide triangular latissimus dorsi muscles angle around the sides of the body toward the spine, under the tapering trapezius muscles. Under these muscles, the rib cage protects the lungs and heart, aorta and vena cava, and pulmonary veins and arteries, which work together to supply essential oxygen-rich blood to the whole body (see figure 9.28). Reiki here also helps any heart or lung condition, from mild to severe.

Client Basic III, Position 4 (Figure 9.29)

Position 4 on the client's back is opposite position 1 on the client's front. To move to this position from position 3, continue to follow the X pattern, moving the hand farthest from you in position 3 close to you, and moving the hand nearest to you in position 3 farther away. Line up your hands, with fingers closed and thumbs touching palms, across the client's back.

The latissimus dorsi and trapezius muscles, the rib cage, the back wall of the diaphragm, the adrenals, and the kidneys receive direct benefit of the Reiki energy in this position. Less directly, the spleen, stomach, and liver are likely to receive the energy. This is the position of choice to focus treatment on any kidney disease or dysfunction, although it should be remembered that the kidneys move up and down with respiration and so may need to be treated in lower positions as well.

Thorough attention to your hands while treating the client in Basic I should result in an easy, quick treatment of the back from this position downward. All of the areas treated will have already received Reiki energy from the front and should still be quite charged with the energy and ready to accomplish the work of accelerated healing.

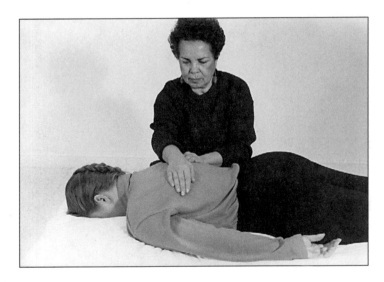

Figure 9.29

This is the position of choice to use informally, in the event of an emergency. While regular attention to the adrenal glands helps them to remain healthy and strong, enabling us to cope with the stresses of daily life, these endocrine system organs are also involved in triggering shock when accidental injury, loss, or trauma occurs. This physiological response is marked by slower heart rate, weak pulse, lower blood pressure, shallow breathing, and cooler body temperature—all indicative of a lower and less stable energetic state.

Once shock sets in, a person responds more slowly to medical care and is less likely to recover completely. It is for this reason that emergency medicine technicians are trained to offer some immediate on-the-scene medical care and to speed the patient to the nearest hospital or trauma center via ambulance or helicopter. The first hour after someone suffers accidental injury is so critical to the success of treatment that emergency medicine professionals call it "the golden hour."

If you are first to arrive at the scene of an accident or disaster, call 911, then perform appropriate first aid, as recommended by the American Red Cross, or administer medical care, but only if you have been trained and are fully qualified and currently certified to do so. If you have no first aid or medical training, make that phone call or find another way to get help. Then, without moving the accident victim, you may bring some comfort by touching the person's shoulder, holding his hand, or placing your hands on the back, or on the abdomen, where the energy can penetrate to the adrenals. This may delay or prevent the onset of shock, extending that window of time when the human body quickly rallies in response to emergency care. If you are unable to reach the person, stand back, raise your hands up, and beam Reiki energy. This, too, will provide some healing.

Continuing the Back: Position 5 (Figure 9.30)

Position 5 on the client's back is opposite position 2 on the client's front, just above the waist. To move to this position from position 5, repeat the X pattern, moving the hand nearest to you in position 4 diagonally across the client's back so that it rests beside the hand furthest from you in position 4. Then move the hand furthest from you in position 4 diagonally toward you, so that it is aligned with the hand above. Fingers should be closed and thumbs touching palms.

The latissimus dorsi muscle stretches from the spine over the soft tissue of the kidneys, pancreas, spleen, liver, and stomach at this level. Although it is unlikely that much energy will be needed here for the gastrointestinal tract organs, if this is a sequential step in a complete treatment and the need for healing of these organs has already been addressed from the front, diabetics and those who have gall bladder problems may well draw strongly here. Simple muscle tension in this area, which is structurally maintained more by muscle than by bone, can be relieved substantially by Reiki hands.

Continuing the Back: Position 6 (Figure 9.31)

This position, on an adult client of average height, parallels position 3 on the client's front, over the waistline. To get into this position, use the X pattern again. Move the hand furthest from you in position 5 diagonally across the client's back so that it rests comfortably beside the hand closest to you in position 5. Then move the hand closest to you in position 5 diagonally away from you, so that it is aligned with the hand below. Keep fingers together and thumbs tucked against palms, and continue to leave a space for the spine.

At the waistline, a diamond-shaped band of muscle called the lumbodorsal fascia connects the latissimus dorsi on the sides of the body to the gluteus medius and gluteus maximus muscles below. The pelvis cradles the intestines in this space. The aorta and the vena cava both divide into smaller circulatory

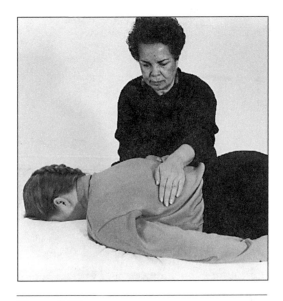

Figure 9.30

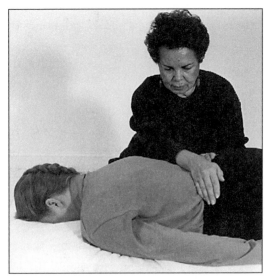

Figure 9.31

channels (called the common iliac artery and the common iliac vein) that carry blood to and from the legs and feet. If there is a substantial draw in this area, muscle tension is the most likely cause.

Continuing the Back: Position 7 (Figure 9.32)

Basic III, position 7 on an adult client of average height, usually spans the lower back, over the top of the pelvis and the sacrum. Unlike the last position on the client's front, this does not require angling the hands into a V. Instead, simply continue to use the X pattern to move from position 6 to position 7, moving the hand nearest to you further away and the hand furthest from you close to you, and moving both downward the width of a hand-span. Keep fingers close together and thumbs against palms, so the aligned hands form a wide band across the client's lower back.

Here stiff muscles sometimes ask for attention. Impaired or blocked nerve pathways from the sacrum or pelvis to the abdomen and extremities can also set off an alarm-bell level of energy activity in Reiki hands. Gastrointestinal disorders and menstrual cramps will also create a strong draw here. Still, if this is the last standard hand position in the sequence of a complete treatment on a client in good health, the amount of time you actually spend sending energy into these areas is not likely to be long.

Extra hand positions are of as much benefit to a client as they are to you during self-treatment. While the client's time constraints must be respected,

Figure 9.32

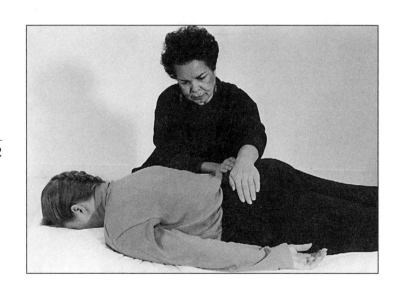

certain extra positions are of such benefit that they should be included whenever time allows. If time is short and only one or two can be fit in, the "tailbone T" (page 169) and the soles of the feet (page 172) are excellent choices.

OPTIONAL POSITIONS

Sciatic Nerves (Figure 9.33)

Treating a client who complains of sharp, shooting pains across the lower back and down the legs requires that you work from each side of the table, in turn. Stand at the client's right side and place your right hand flat across the right hip, about halfway out from center. Beneath your right hand and perpendicular to it, at the level of the wrist, lay your left hand down on the side of the client's lower buttock, over the gluteus medius muscle. Allow the Reiki energy to penetrate, stabilize in intensity, and then diminish before moving to the other side of the table.

Now standing at the client's left side, place your left hand flat across the hip, as before. Beneath your left hand and perpendicular to it at the wrist, lay your right hand down on the side of the client's lower buttock. As usual, allow the energy to flow through at least one full healing cycle.

This is an extra position, requested most often by people who have sciatica, a catch-all term for inflammation or damage to the sciatic nerve bundles, which exit from the lumbar spine and sacrum and then travel into the lower limbs. By

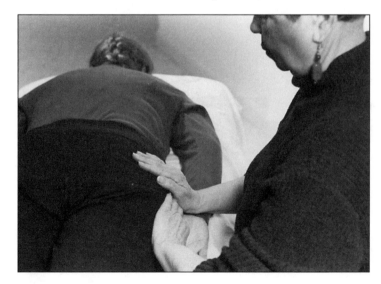

Figure 9.33

applying your hands in the L-shaped position described above, you address the need for sciatic nerve healing at its source, even though the pain may be felt at some distance: in the groin, the thighs, the knees, the shins and calves, the ankles, or the feet. Unless there is a separate injury to one of these sites, which has caused localized pain, Reiki hands applied in this position will generally provide relief from sciatica and its myriad symptoms. Since problems in this area are often chronic, expect to do repeated treatments before lasting relief is obtained.

COMPLETING THE TREATMENT

Just as there are many reasons to start a treatment on the upper back, so there are many reasons to continue the treatment down to the lower back, and to conclude the treatment with both hands in a T formation over the sacrum and coccyx. However, some clients prefer a treatment that ends with a hand on the back of the neck and a hand across the sacrum, for balancing the energy flow throughout the torso. Others enjoy a treatment that ends with both hands flat on the soles of the feet, for grounding before they sit up and get down from the table.

Tailbone T (Figure 9.34)
One way to close a complete Reiki treatment on a client is the "tailbone T," which sends energy deep into the sacrum and coccyx, targeting the colon and the rectum, as well as all the nerves that exit from the sacrum and coccyx and travel down the legs to the toes. This position is easy to do: while standing at the side of the table, place one hand horizontally across the client's lower back, covering the sacrum, and the other hand perpendicular to the first, covering the coccyx, so that your hands form a T. The client is clothed, so allow any sense of awkwardness that you feel to dissolve, because the benefits of healing in this area can be remarkable. Let any resistance you feel give way to compassion.

None of us learns to walk without falling, and some people, particularly skaters, skiers, and martial artists, endure many falls in the course of normal training. Because of this, Reiki hands applied over the tailbone can be immensely comforting. Although an injury may be many years old and apparently healed, the trauma may not be completely released, and so the body will hold the impact in its cellular memory, affecting the health of the tissues in the area. Reiki hands can effectively reach back in time to the original injury and sense of trauma, allowing the body to complete the necessary healing and be fully healthy now. Healing such an old injury may require several treatment sessions.

Another reason to focus on this area to finish a treatment is that many adults suffer from hemorrhoids, which cause mild to severe discomfort, depending upon the degree of neglect or attention that has been given them. In particular, women who are pregnant or who have been recently pregnant often suffer physical stress on the tissues in this area. Aging adults, especially those who are sedentary or who do not eat well, can suffer hemorrhoids as well. Since these tears in the lining of the rectum and colon can progress to the stage where surgery is required, Reiki hands applied here can provide preventive maintenance.

My teacher, Rev. Beth Gray, felt strongly that this position was an excellent way to end a treatment, but during my own years of teaching Reiki, I have had students ask for an alternative position that felt less invasive of privacy. The following two positions are good alternatives; I also encourage students to do both these positions in order to close. The first position is a wonderful way to encourage the energy to flow in rhythm with the natural pulsing of the cerebrospinal fluid through the spine. This supports a sense of centeredness and balance. The second position draws the energy down into the legs all the way to the soles of the feet, so it is grounding. Clients who get up from the table feeling centered, balanced, and grounded, as well as peaceful and relaxed, and have high praise for Reiki!

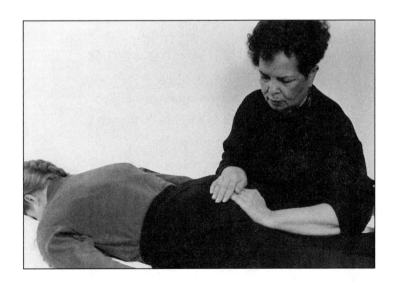

Figure 9.34

Cervical Vertebrae and Sacrum (Figure 9.35)

This position makes an excellent close to a complete treatment of the back, as it covers the cervical vertebrae of the neck—an area not addressed by the standard positions—and the sacrum, just below the lumbar vertebrae of the lower back (Position 7). As your hands span the length of the client's spine, from top to bottom, the energy flows not only directly under your hands, but radiates between and outward from them in a way that feels both balancing and grounding. Whether this is a result of the energy following the spinal cord and the nerve pathways that exit from the vertebrae or of the use of a more subtle anatomy, such as the energy meridians described in Chinese medicine or the chakra system described in Kundalini yoga, makes no difference: the soothing, centering effect is something clients enjoy.

Treatment of the neck can bring respite from muscle tension, headaches, neuralgia, and herpes simplex outbreaks in or on the mouth or nose; treatment of the sacrum soothes nerve pathways leading from this bony structure to the abdominal organs, and down the legs, front and back, all the way to the feet. Treating both areas at once can provide relief for more serious conditions affecting the cerebrospinal fluid, the spinal cord, or the spine itself. If your client has suffered spinal cord injury, remind him that repeated treatments can play a key role in recovery; also remember that allowing your hands to remain in position through several repetitions of the energy-flow cycle to deepen healing can be very effective in accelerating the process.

Figure 9.35

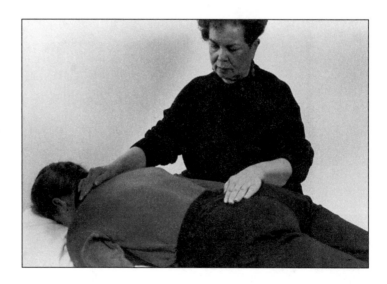

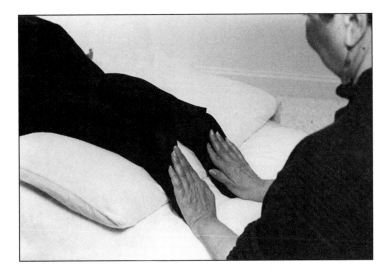

Figure 9.36

Soles of the Feet (Figure 9.36)

Reflexologists will tell you that the soles of the feet map, in miniature, the rest of the body: the big toes of each foot correspond to the head, the eyes, the pineal and pituitary glands, and the mouth and sinuses; the balls of the feet correspond to the upper chest, and include the bronchi, the lungs, and the breasts; and so on. Whether or not this is true, Reiki on the soles of the feet certainly can be felt at other locations in the body and is extremely relaxing. Perhaps most important of all, Reiki hands applied here have the effect of drawing the healing energy now concentrated in the torso into the extremities. This is both balancing and grounding for the client, who is about to be roused for the final time, given only a few moments to return to normal awareness, and then sent on his way to home or to work and the demands of daily life.

Perhaps the best way to decide how you would like to end your client treatments is to have a fellow Reiki practitioner exchange sessions with you, and sample the effects of the energy in each of these positions. You might also offer a client the same opportunity at his initial treatment session, and then work according to his preference at subsequent sessions.

As with all hand positions, listen to your hands to determine the moment to shift to the next position, and—in this case—to conclude the treatment.

However informal or formal your session has been, ask the client to come back to normal awareness gradually, and to take his time in getting up into a sitting position (as he may feel lightheaded from positional blood pressure change or disoriented from having been asleep and dreaming). If possible, offer him a glass of cool spring water. The sensation of sipping and drinking cool water in a relaxed state is centering. Return eyeglasses if they have been taken off for the treatment. Put shoes close by as well. Encourage your client to step off the table only when he feels ready. Thank him for the opportunity to offer him Reiki healing, and invite him to give you a call in a day or two if he has comments he would like to share or questions he would like to ask. Then see him to the door to say good-bye.

Chances are you will feel energized and relaxed yourself, and if you catch a glimpse of yourself in the mirror, you will be surprised by your own radiance— all aftereffects of working with the Reiki energy, which is intent on healing you, too! Enjoy the sensations of energy flow, heightened sensory awareness, mental clarity, peace of mind, and wearing a smile that begins in your heart. Just listen to your hands. The energy flowing through them will teach you what you need to know.

10

COMPLETING THE
REIKI I CLASS

After hours of hands-on practice and discussion of the practicalities of Reiki as a career choice, students are sometimes surprised to realize that they have still one more attunement to receive. This fourth and final attunement of a traditional Usui Reiki class is done by the teacher in the same way as the earlier attunements, yet it has a markedly different effect. It completes the sequence, stabilizing the channel of healing within each Reiki practitioner so that it is set to last a lifetime.

"I feel good." A smile. A nod. "Really good. And my hands feel really hot."
"My hands feel like there's a magnet between them, holding them together—and as if there are currents of energy flowing all around them. Neat."
"My heart feels more open. I want to laugh and cry at the same time."
"I saw that swirling royal purple color again. My hands feel the same pulsing—just more intense."
"Hmmm. . . . This is hard to describe. My hands are very tingly. I think if I waved my hands through the air right now, they would leave a trail of tiny lights."

"Peaceful. My hands are on. There's a sort of throbbing between my palms. And that's all I feel."

In addition to stabilizing the channel, the fourth attunement also seals the Reiki practitioner so that he need not take on another person's pain or suffering in order to help that person heal. Years of experience have taught me that this sealing process works in the other direction as well. A client given a Reiki treatment by a practitioner who is himself ill, or simply in a negative frame of mind, will not pick up the practitioner's illness or negativity. Instead, the Reiki energy will assist them both in their healing as it courses through the hands of the practitioner to the client.

The traditional sequence of four attunements establishes the ability to channel Reiki energy at a threshold below the level of conscious intention. Many practitioners trained in this way experience their hands turning on spontaneously as they walk along a crowded city sidewalk, sit at a computer writing a letter to a friend, or watch flashes of lightning during a storm. Their hands may even turn on as they sleep.

The sense of being in harmony with life, which we all experience at times, is highlighted through the attunements for the conscious mind to see. The soul absorbs the lesson that this harmony with the universal life force is both natural and constant; the body, transformed, supports this lesson so that mind and heart can appreciate this spiritual truth, enjoy the feeling of flow, and gradually be healed of thoughts of separation and isolation, and know joy.

REIKI'S PLACE IN YOUR LIFE: A PREVIEW

Before the Reiki master brings the class to a close and gives you your certificate, she is likely to describe for you how your life might change as a result of your decision to learn Reiki. While some of these changes are as simple and natural as feeling a sense of greater well-being—and as easy to accept—others are not. Friends and family members may come to see you in a new light. Companions who do not have your best interests at heart may drift away, freeing you to become involved in healthier, happier relationships. Work assignments that do not support you on all levels may end gradually or abruptly, offering you the chance to make new career choices that are more rewarding.

As you continue to treat yourself daily with Reiki, you will find that you can cope with such changes. Yet your Reiki master may still encourage you to stay in touch, to visit a Reikishare (healing circle) or two, to make some "Reiki friends," and to consider assisting at future Reiki I classes, all with the goal of supporting you as a new practitioner and helping you to discover that you have an opportunity to become a part of a local and global community of like-minded people committed to Reiki healing. She may even describe, in some detail, how to establish a professional Reiki practice. While this may seem an unlikely career move to you as you complete your Reiki I class, listen well to your teacher's advice: she has already made this transition, and she is well aware of the business and legal requirements of this profession. This information can help you decide whether or not this is an opportunity you might eventually want to pursue.

REIKI LEVEL I CERTIFICATION

Completing a traditional Reiki level I class marks a joyful moment in time that opens up infinite possibilities, literally and figuratively. The experience of your hands is one of conscious union with the universal life-force energy. You may ride the flow of this energy to miracles, as well as to greater day-to-day peace of mind.

This moment is marked with a ceremony in which your teacher presents you with a signed, dated, and sealed certificate, charged with healing energy, acknowledging that you have completed the basic course in the Usui Reiki method of natural healing. As you thank your teacher, your fellow students may applaud you, and someone may even snap your picture. (Don't be photo-shy. If your teacher would like your picture, it will be so that she has a record that she and others may use to send distant healing to you at your request.) With your Reiki I certificate, you are qualified to practice Reiki professionally.* While you may never set up a professional practice, the pleasure of working with Reiki to heal and create positive changes will bring you soul satisfaction.

---

*Please check local and state regulations regarding the practice of holistic health care in your location. Make a trip to your local borough, town, or city hall to inquire about necessary business permits; see appendix 3 for more information on how to contact state regulatory agencies.

THE FIRST FEW DAYS AFTER THE REIKI CLASS

Once you have completed the Reiki class, you might think that your spiritual adventure is at an end. In fact, your path still stretches out before you, now even more brightly illuminated: you can look for more clarity of purpose, easier focus on your goals, a strong sense of being guided, and more frequent synchronicities—that which is right for you appearing at just the perfect time. However, the most obvious abilities that you will be developing as an outcome of the class are intuition and a heightening of your "inner senses"—correlates of the external senses—which allow you to perceive information transmitted via the flow of Reiki through your hands into the physical body and the energy field around the body (the human aura). Through this heightened awareness, you may learn to understand more about the holistic nature of healing and come to appreciate the powerful impact of a positive attitude on health and well-being.

During the days immediately following your class your hands are likely to feel quite active. You may experience some surprising sensations; you may also be awakened from deep sleep by the feeling of the energy flowing through them. If this happens, just put your hands to use: lay them over your heart or gently rest them against your spouse's shoulders. The flow of the energy will bring healing even as you fall back to sleep.

Also, if you do the hand positions for self-treatment before you get out of bed in the morning, don't be surprised if you discover reddened handprints on yourself when you are in the shower. Your circulation has been stimulated by the flow of Reiki energy. Although these marks may seem a little alarming, only good has been done; they will gradually fade within a few hours.

You may also discover that your hands turn on at odd times. You may be in the middle of giving a big presentation at work, holding a pointer to a flip chart, and suddenly you will feel the flow of Reiki energy. Or you might be playing with your nine-month-old baby, trying to get him to take his favorite stuffed toy, when you notice your hands are on. Or you might be spooning soup into a bowl at a shelter for the homeless, when you realize that your hands are suddenly very warm.

All of these events are ongoing lessons in the constant presence of Spirit guiding the healing energy into all aspects of your life, and through you into the lives of everyone with whom you come in contact who needs healing. As you realize this is occurring, you will find ways to invite the energy to join in. When you sit down to dinner you might hold your Reiki hands over your food—to boost its healthy nutritional value—and discover that this feels like a blessing, a way of saying grace. Or you may go to the garden store, pick out some packets of seeds, and realize that they will grow more quickly into beautiful healthy plants if you spend a little time charging them with Reiki. Or you might decide that if you have to change the bandages every day over a cut that took stitches, you might as well send a little Reiki into the tape and gauze, as well as into the cut. And your impulse will be right: experienced Reiki practitioners will tell you that these are all effective ways to expand the benefits of Reiki energy in your life.

You will also find yourself "volunteered" to give the support that Reiki can provide. You might be half-dozing, watching TV, your hands limp in your lap, when your dog nuzzles you and then shoves his head under your hands. Or a friend might call and ask if you would be willing to go with her to visit her mother in the hospital. Or a fellow student in a karate class might take a bad fall, retreat to the sidelines, and ask if there is anything anyone can do to relieve the pain of his sprained ankle until the ice and aspirin start to take effect.

Saying "yes" to using your hands for healing ought to be easy, don't you think? Many times, it is. You reach out a hand and someone takes it. You ask, "Can I help?" and are beckoned closer. At first, though, offering to use Reiki on a friend or family member who needs healing may seem like the last thing you want to do. Here is someone who loves you, who knows your faults as well as your strengths. What will you do or say if instead of accepting your kind offer, your best friend rolls her eyes heavenward and says, "Oh, don't tell me you're into that New Age stuff. . . ."

You'll soon discover that your ego and your spirit can survive skepticism unscathed, and that the healing energy in your hands is not affected by other people's opinions. While this is a comfort, there will still come a time when you will want to put this experience into words and are uncertain how to begin.

The easiest way to describe Reiki is in terms of experiences that are already familiar, such as massage or other forms of bodywork. However, if your friend is willing to accept the comfort of your touch without any preliminary explanation, the sensations of the Reiki energy flow that your friend registers may suggest comfortable comparisons to him. You might hear him say, "Your hands feel like a heating pad" as you place them over an old injury, or "like an ice pack" over a more recent muscle pull or tear.

One of my students, a college professor and department chairperson, learned Reiki after coming regularly for treatments for three years. I asked him if he planned to tell his wife.

"Well, I haven't gotten around to it just yet."

"Don't you find that you want to use it to help her with her migraines?" I asked.

"I do use it. Kind of. I ask her if she would like me to rub her neck, and then I put my hands on her shoulders and just let the energy flow."

I couldn't help laughing. "Don't you think she's figured out by now that you aren't really rubbing her neck?"

"I'm sure she has, but I think she doesn't mind. She knows that whatever I'm doing feels good and takes away her headaches."

Even with gentle encouragement, this man has not been able to talk to his wife about Reiki, perhaps because he feels that doing so might threaten his marriage. And indeed there are even people who refuse to learn Reiki at all unless their spouses do so at the same time. They want nothing to occur in their lives that might potentially upset their partner.

People who are in such self-described "rock solid" traditional marriages often have carefully built their shared lives. Yet sometimes they need to remind themselves that a good marriage is strong enough to support the growth of both individuals without endangering the love they have for each other.

Reiki can be that reminder. Many couples discover that after one of them learns Reiki they have a new kind of touch—a very tender and comforting touch—to share with one another. Even when one partner chooses to learn and the other does not, the energy works to support their unconditional love for each other, as well as their personal health and the health of their families. Often the resistant partner decides, in time, to learn Reiki as well, on the basis of the evidence before his eyes: a healthier, happier spouse and a renewed sense of vitality in his own body following treatment with Reiki.

It is rare but not unheard of that Reiki may also quicken the dissolution of a marriage already in crisis, in which the partners have been at odds for some time and are only growing farther apart. Hands-on and distant healing with Reiki can lessen the emotional pain of loss and speed personal recovery for both partners; the flow of the energy also provides a good foundation for former marriage partners to remain lifelong friends.

For the most part, however, as Reiki speeds your spiritual growth all those around you will feel a little more love and light, and pick up their own pace of growth to keep company with you. New friends who are aware, sensitive, and gently loving will find you as well, sometimes from halfway across the world, and they will not seem "new" at all but as familiar to you as if they had journeyed with you lifetime after lifetime, and are only now coming home again to your heart.

Perhaps that is the way of it: You bring Reiki home, whether you speak of it or not, by your own lighted presence. Those around you feel and accept and celebrate the change in you—or else they leave—and others find their way to your side, smiling. You find you feel safe, secure, and content wherever you are, in the flow of unconditional love through your hands. One day you realize you are "home," and you know you live in your heart.

ESTABLISHING A SUPPORT NETWORK

Today there are many Reiki masters teaching publicly and privately all over the world: announcements of classes are made in the calendar sections of city newspapers; healing-circle and Reikishare dates are posted on websites; Reiki practitioners' business cards pepper bookstore and health-food store bulletin boards and even the bulletin boards in some medical practitioners' offices.

Meeting other Reiki practitioners to share experiences and exchange treatments has never been easier. Still, some of your best Reiki friends may be people you met in your Reiki class. If you feel an immediate connection to someone in your class, let them know. Exchange phone numbers. Get your new friend's e-mail address if he has one. Or make a date to get together in a few weeks to practice on each other, and then continue to meet to exchange treatments on a regular basis. You will discover that it is wonderful to have someone in your life who understands what you are talking about when you describe the energy in your hands and your experiences with Reiki.

There is also great benefit in being able to ask questions and get answers after the class is over. A healing circle or Reikishare can give you this opportunity; so can access to the Internet. For example, in a recent posting to a Reiki mailing list, a practitioner in Italy asked about working on an elderly friend who had osteoarthritis. Within a few days, a practitioner from Canada and a Reiki master from Holland had responded with descriptions of their experiences and some very specific suggestions about the frequency of treatments needed for this chronic condition.

There is also a lot of pleasure in being able to "send postcards" via the Internet, marking your progress to someone who also appreciates the journey. As your own health improves, and your spiritual growth accelerates, talking with a Reiki friend can make you feel as charged up with the comforting, healing energy as doing an actual treatment on a client.

Ideally your Reiki master will also be able to provide you with some support after the class is over, even if only in the form of occasional telephone conversations to answer your questions as they arise. Although many travel to teach, and have busy, complicated schedules, some host regular healing circles in their homes. Most Reiki masters are happy to have you return to assist at a Reiki class and will invite you to do so at the conclusion of level I, so that you may share your Reiki stories and the lessons of your experiences may be learned by all.

ASSISTING AT A LEVEL I CLASS

Whenever your teacher schedules a class in your area, you can take advantage of her invitation to assist at the class. You will probably share stories of your experiences with Reiki, which add to the beautiful, kaleidoscopic effect of hearts being repatterned by healing hands. You might also guide a student who feels like he is "all thumbs" through the hand positions. In assisting your teacher you will receive as much—and more—than you contribute. You will review the Reiki teachings, get the opportunity to ask questions and receive answers, and have the chance to see former classmates and make new friends. Perhaps most important, the energy of Reiki will be charging the very air you breathe with light and unconditional love. When the class is over you will find that you feel clear and sharp and energized—or quietly rested and restored—whatever is most healing for you at the time.

ESTABLISHING A PROFESSIONAL PRACTICE

A surprising number of Reiki practitioners eventually become part-time or full-time professional practitioners, so your Reiki master is likely to give you an overview of the requirements for establishing a professional practice. She may begin by encouraging you with this bit of good news: once you make a commitment to treating Reiki clients on a regular basis, you will discover that the universe readily sends what you need your way—from an appropriate space to steady clients. In order to call forth this support, however, you will need to make good use of the resources available to you at every stage of the transition from your old to your new career. This is a beautiful and loving expression of your intention, to which the universe will respond in kind.

This may mean that you clear out a spare bedroom or finish the basement to turn it into a treatment room—an investment of time, energy, and a bit of hard work. Or it may mean sacrificing your weekly dinner out for a while in order to put aside a small amount from each paycheck to pay for a bodywork table. You may give up a few weekends to take a class in accounting, or spend several evenings reading books about how to start and run a small business. Whatever it takes to establish your professional practice in your community, from getting required business permits and liability insurance to keeping fresh flowers in the treatment room, be willing to make the effort and expend the necessary time, energy, and money. Balance your enthusiasm for this career change with conscientious and responsible planning, and then be a reliable service provider as well as an inspired Reiki healing practitioner. In this way, you can "do an honest day's work"—and enjoy doing the work you love.

Selecting a Treatment Table

When you decide that you are ready to buy a bodywork table, shop around to get the table you want for the best price. You can visit retail stores that sell massage and bodywork tables exclusively and "try out" the merchandise. You might also find a good table, complete with headrest, bolsters, and case, at a discount ware-house store, such as Sam's Club, Costco, or B.J.'s. These outlets do not stock a wide variety, but their products are very reasonably priced. If you feel comfortable shopping online, browse the Internet to discover many more sources—and don't forget to pick up a copy of the latest alternative health or New Age magazines in your health food store. These publications often list directories of suppliers in their pages, as well as publishing paid ads (also see the resources list in appendix 3). Occasionally it is possible to buy a used table from a massage therapist retiring from practice or returning to school to study for a different profession.

A good massage table will be adjustable to your height (and will also have enough range to accommodate the height of the people in your life who would like to work on you). Ideally you should be able to stand or sit at the side, head, or foot of the table in a balanced and relaxed posture; you should also be able to place your hands on a client in the standard positions without discomfort or strain. Most adjustable tables can be set at heights from 22 to 30 inches.

The surface of the table should be vinyl or another sturdy fabric that is easy to wipe clean. Soft padding under this surface adds to the client's comfort—and the thicker the padding, the greater the level of comfort. (You can also soften a too-firm table surface by covering it with a comforter or feather bed underneath a sheet.)

Some tables are designed with an opening to allow clients to rest their heads without stressing the vertebrae of the neck; more commonly, table manu-facturers include a padded headrest (or offer one for an additional fee) that can be fitted into holes at one end of the table. Although you may initially resist the idea of any extra expense, most clients prefer headrest support when receiving bodywork, because it allows them to relax more deeply. For this reason, you may quickly discover this is an important and worthwhile purchase.

Some massage tables are not portable. Unless you are completely settled and know that you will always practice in one particular treatment room (say, in a chiropractor's office), get a portable table that folds in half and has collaps-ible legs of wood or metal. This will allow you to take advantage of invitations to healing circles, to provide in-home care for those who are elderly or too ill to come to your location, and to volunteer to meet runners at the race's end with a smile and an offer of Reiki healing.

The weight and folded dimensions of the massage table should also be a consideration. If you are of slight build yourself, you do not want to have to haul a heavy table around with you. Extremely light tables sell at a premium, however, so if possible, test height and weight before making your purchase. You may also need to make sure that the final folded dimensions of the massage table will allow you to conveniently carry it in the hatch, trunk, or backseat of your car.

Finally, investing in a cover for your massage table is a good idea. Not only does a cover offer some protection to your table as it travels with you, it also provides protection at home from dust, dirt, ordinary knocks, and—perhaps most important—from cats, who seem to prefer a massage table steeped in loving energy as a scratching post over almost anything else.

Setting Up a Treatment Room

Once you have purchased a massage or bodywork table and committed to taking care of it, you will find that you begin to attract friends, family members, and clients (referred to you by word-of-mouth or responding to your advertising) with more frequency. As they come to you, you will want to present as professional an image as possible.

Create a waiting area that is clean, comfortable, peaceful, and convenient to your treatment room and a restroom. As for the treatment room itself, once you have dedicated it to its new purpose, all evidence of its former existence as a back office or spare bedroom should be removed, including the phone. Furnish it simply, and keep it clean and uncluttered. Your treatment table should be the main focus. Rely on soft lighting, preferably on a dimmer switch, to make this space even more conducive to deep relaxation.

In addition to your treatment table, you will probably want to have a cabinet or wide shelf that can hold clean sheets, pillows, pillowcases, a comforter or quilt, and extra pillows or a bolster. A table to hold a pitcher of spring water and drinking glasses for you and your client is a good idea. A glasses' rest for eyeglasses is a thoughtful touch. Keep your calendar or appointment book, and your business cards readily available to make it easier for you and your client to schedule a next appointment.

You might also accessorize this room with items not so much of practical value as of personal style: plants, music, a rocking chair in the corner, books on alternative medicine, pottery, paintings, photographs, aromatherapy candles, incense. In making such choices, consider your client's comfort first. (For example, out of respect for the comfort of a regular client who is an allergy-sufferer, you might choose not to use aromatherapy or incense in this room, and to keep it off limits from pets. On the other hand, if you are trained in aromatherapy and want to augment the energy of Reiki with healing scents, you might simply decide to air out the room by opening a window before a client who is an allergy-sufferer comes for a treatment.)

Whatever you decide, enjoy the process of creating a healing space for yourself and others. Use the room and the resources within it with gratitude and love. Frame and display your Reiki certificate on the wall, for it clearly states your professional qualifications to your clients and carries the charge of the Reiki energy. Your Reiki master has signed, sealed, and attuned the certificate—and given it to you—with love.

Record Keeping

Like any small-business professional, you must keep good records for tax purposes. While an appointment book may be sufficient for your needs, the IRS prefers to see a log of actual time spent engaged in client services. In addition, a ledger of income (cash, check, or barter received) and expenses incurred is also necessary. Remember that the IRS is particularly stringent about deductions for home offices. Review the requirements for legitimate deductions each year, and provide careful and methodical documentation for any that you claim. If you are in any doubt as to how to do your tax return as a part-time or full-time self-employed alternative healing practitioner, use the services of a reputable certified public accountant (CPA) to ensure that the information you provide to the government about your profession is accurate and complete.

In addition to keeping records for tax purposes, it is also good business practice to keep confidential client files. While you are not legally obligated to make notes on your client's progress at the end of each treatment session, you may find that such records are of value to you and to your client in understanding the process of recovery, clarifying personal and professional goals, and deciding on lifestyle changes.

Another essential is business liability insurance. This is available through bodywork and massage therapy professional associations, as well as through the International Association of Reiki Professionals (see appendix 3 for contact details for specific organizations). Getting and maintaining liability insurance will allow you to treat clients professionally at a wellness center, in a hospital, in a school, or at home—so long as you identify the facility to your insurer as a "co-insured." If you are a homeowner, you may also discover that you need a modification or addendum to your homeowner's insurance policy. Don't resist doing this paperwork. It helps to ensure that your business practice meets all legal requirements. This is a simple way to practice the fourth Reiki principle in your workplace: do your best; act with integrity. That creates an intangible value that your clients will appreciate and that you will experience as greater peace of mind.

Once you have succeeded in making the career change to professional practitioner, you may wonder if the happiness you feel in doing work that you love is too good to last. Trust that it can. Right work, in harmony with spiritual purpose and in service to humankind, has a way of supporting a person in quiet contentment and joy.

CREATING THE LIFE YOU WANT WITH REIKI

After the Reiki I class, allow yourself the possibility of growth in whatever way you are guided: learn other healing modalities; combine them with Reiki practice; volunteer to work with AIDs patients; take Reiki "on the road," providing relaxation breaks as an alternative to coffee breaks in corporations; start a spiritual studies group; volunteer at an animal shelter or wildlife refuge; work as a chef and Reiki every ingredient you use in your recipes; create a garden where every plant is charged with Reiki energy and the show of beauty dazzles the eye and comforts the soul; write to your town councilmen and your mayor, or write to your congressmen about your community concerns and Reiki the stationery, the stamp, and every word. Let yourself be inspired, drawn by love in new directions. Come into a relationship with yourself that is healing to the whole world.

REIKI LEVEL II
AND BEYOND

No book, however complete, can provide you the same benefit as attending a class, because a book cannot empower you with the Reiki energy to be a channel for healing. This is true whether you are interested in learning the basic, advanced, or master course in the Usui Reiki method of natural healing. Being properly attuned by a trained and certified Reiki master is necessary to accomplish this transformation.

Because this is true, and because the methods of distant healing taught in traditional Reiki level II classes are so varied—and valid—what follows should be considered only as a broad overview of the concepts involved and in no way a substitute for the specific instructional content a Reiki master provides in class, or for the in-depth discussions he leads.

This overview of concepts discussed in a traditional Reiki level II class will seem most accessible to a reader who has already completed Reiki level I and reads this in anticipation of further training, or to a reader who has already completed Reiki level II and reads this as a review. Without a solid foundation of practical experience with hands-on Reiki, the reader may find his imagination stretched beyond his conscious mind's ability to believe. Any reader who is in this position is advised to receive a Reiki treatment or take a level I class before continuing further.

During a traditional Reiki distant-healing class, which usually takes place over at least two to two and a half days, the practitioner receives two or three additional attunements that further increase his ability to channel the healing energy and expand his perceptions of the energy's subtle flow; he is taught how to draw three symbols and how to use them with hands-on and distant-healing treatments; and he is taught a method of distant healing. When he has completed the class, he receives a certificate of completion of training in the "advanced course in the Reiki Method of Natural Healing."

As a result of the variety of attunements, symbols, and distant-healing methods taught by Hawayo Takata to the twenty-two Reiki masters she initiated, what you are taught by your traditional Reiki master in a level II class may be quite different from what is touched on here. Trust that the energy is powerful enough to work through many methods, many symbols, many hands, many teachers, with unconditional love. Trust also that you as a Reiki practitioner are guided to learn in whatever way is best for you, and that your level II class will mark the beginning of a much deeper level of experience for you, not with a hard and fast dividing line, but with the gentleness and gradualness of awakening to a new and beautiful vision of your world.

11

REIKI LEVEL II: AN OVERVIEW OF THE ADVANCED COURSE

You may have discovered that the delightful "electricity" you feel in your hands charges and energizes you so effectively that you simply want more. You may have become intrigued by the idea of an easier way to send healing energy to your back than by the standard hands-on positions, and decided that whatever it is, you have to learn it. Or you may have been so happily surprised by the positive changes that unfolded in your professional and personal lives when you learned Reiki I that you are eager to take the next class. All of these are excellent reasons to learn Reiki level II, the distant-healing method. And there is another: if Reiki I introduced you to a depth of spiritual experience that you never felt before, you may have come to love the practice of Reiki and may feel a kind of spiritual longing to learn more.

For most people, though, the desire to learn Reiki distance healing is sparked by a single confrontation with the limits of their current practical knowledge: someone emotionally close but physically hundreds of miles away needs healing, and short of dropping everything and getting on a plane to be at that person's bedside, there is nothing you can do but pray. While prayer can and does work miracles, when you are aware that the touch of your Reiki hands can go a long way in the same direction, it is natural to want to add to your prayers the power of the healing energy that sees no limits to health.

Whatever your reasons for wanting to learn Reiki distant healing, sometime during the course of your level II class, you are likely to discover that other students have come to learn for reasons much like your own. For most practitioners, the moments just before a Reiki level II class are full of friendly smiles, warm hellos, and anticipation. Yet when the Reiki master invites each practitioner to share an experience with Reiki since learning level I, the stories that are told quickly bring everyone to focused attention.

"What's been going on in your life?" he might ask. "Have you any stories to share about working with hands-on healing?"

> *"The very first time that I used Reiki was on my mother-in-law, who has glaucoma. I asked her to lie down on the couch and to let me put my hands over her eyes. I felt my hands turn on and get really hot and then, after about twenty minutes, they started to cool down. I lifted them up and looked at my mother-in-law and her eyes had actually receded back into the eye sockets, because the pressure inside them had gone down. She said her eyes felt better, but when she looked in the mirror, she couldn't believe it. She could see the difference, too."*

> *"I asked a friend of mine if I could give him a full treatment for a Christmas present. He said sure, but that the only time off he had was on the same afternoon when he had scheduled a massage—that was his Christmas present to himself. I worked on him for about forty-five minutes—he's pretty healthy, so the treatment didn't take long. He said he felt good and he thanked me and went on to his appointment with the massage therapist. Well, he called me later to tell me that the massage therapist had asked him why he had scheduled a treatment. There were no tense muscles, no spasms, no knots. The massage therapist had never worked on anyone who was already so relaxed."*

> *"I am a massage therapist, and what I found is that since learning level I, my*

work is a lot easier. I start a massage now by just placing my hands on the client's shoulders for a couple of minutes and letting the energy flow. I can feel this easing of tension. Then I start the massage. The clients seem to find this really soothing—and I don't have to put as much pressure into the strokes, which is a lot easier on me."

"One of my good friends is an elderly woman who is diabetic. She had some of her toes amputated, so she doesn't get out much. After I learned level I, I was anxious to try Reiki out on her, so I scheduled an appointment to come to visit. She was very open-minded when I explained what I wanted to do—and she was sensitive to the energy. When I was doing the hand positions for Basic I, she said she could feel the energy all the way down into her missing toes."

"One of my daughters had a baby a few months ago, shortly after my level I class. She invited me to be there in the delivery room and work on her back when she was in labor and giving birth. She said it really helped—and it was certainly a joy for me to be present at the birth of my grandson."

"My husband's father is being treated for a cancerous tumor under his sternum. My husband and I are able to visit him at night, so I do Reiki on him then. I've also asked some friends who are level II Reiki channels to send healing, and they have. The doctors say that they're really pleased with the way the tumor's been shrinking. I know that some of that is the result of radiation and chemotherapy, but the doctors say they're surprised there has been so much improvement. So I'm encouraged to learn level II."

SHARING COMMON GROUND, EXPLORING NEW GROUND

Such stories reveal the gentleness and compassion that mark so many Reiki practitioners—and also remind everyone present of all the conditions to which they can apply their Reiki hands. Whatever the practitioners' individual experiences of working with the energy, whatever their occupations, they share their stories now with an appreciation of the Reiki energy's power to heal where hope was slim. In so doing they inspire and learn from each other, strengthening their foundation of understanding with shared insights and their sense of self-acceptance with nonjudgmental and loving attention to their fellow practitioners.

Reiki distant healing enables the Reiki practitioner who has a foundation of experience with hands-on healing to call for an increase in the flow of energy during client- or self-treatment, to address emotional and mental issues requiring healing, and to send the same Spirit-guided universal life-force energy to someone at another point in space and time. Reiki distant healing, also referred to as absentee healing, allows the practitioner to send Reiki to someone who is literally absent—perhaps thousands of miles away from her location. It also allows the practitioner to send Reiki to herself using the same method for the increased healing benefits it provides. This may be as easy to comprehend as the positive effect of saying a prayer for a friend who is anesthetized and undergoing surgery, or for yourself as you are about to make an important change in your life. Or it can seem as mind-boggling and straight out of science fiction as time travel, as it permits the practitioner to send healing into the past (to help recovery from traumatic events) or into the future (to events that are expected to be stressful), apparently without any disruptions in the time continuum at all.

Reiki distant healing is, in many ways, like prayer: it involves a brief ritual, symbolic gestures, words of blessing, and an attitude of surrender to the spiritual intelligence that guides all our lives. Yet it is not prayer as most people think of it, and will work as well for an atheist or an agnostic as it will for a devout Christian or Buddhist or Muslim or Jew.

How does the idea of Reiki distant healing fit with such ease into so many people's spiritual lives? This foundation is laid in learning hands-on Reiki: we are reminded in a way that we can never forget that we are profoundly connected to Spirit. On this foundation we can build a house of the heart that stands high and visible from very far away, brilliant with light from every window and every door, a comfort to both strangers and those closest to us. This comfort is for body, mind, heart, and soul, and can bring the easing of suffering, the calming of mental turmoil, the joy of unconditional love, and strong inner guidance to us and to those who receive the Reiki distant healing, whether they are across the room, across the ocean, or across time.

Yet despite the sense of the sacred that permeates the practice of Reiki distant healing like the scent of a beautiful flower, putting it into practice can seem quite ordinary. Many times a distant healing begins with a practitioner's phone call to a friend, the discovery that the friend is not well, a few kind

192

words of sympathy, and the recognition that something can be done to help. Instead of saying only, "Gosh, I wish you felt better" before getting off the phone, the Reiki practitioner can be a lot more upbeat; he can add, "I'm going to sit down right now and send you some healing energy. You just get some rest. I'll talk to you soon." A phone call a few hours or a few days later will find the friend feeling better; this will be no surprise to the Reiki practitioner, who has learned from experience the effectiveness of the distant-healing method.

WORKING WITH SYMBOLS

Imagine being able to send a message that actually makes the person who receives it feel better. Possible? Certainly. You send messages like that every day—when you mail your friend a birthday card, or you pick up the phone to congratulate your son on his promotion, or you have a singing telegram delivered to your wife to celebrate your anniversary. Now imagine being able to send such messages without using the services of the post office or the phone company. Instead of writing a letter, addressing an envelope, putting the letter in the envelope, sealing the envelope closed, licking a stamp, and setting the stamp down in the proper place, what might you do? How could you connect to someone far away? Even using the telephone requires you to key in a series of numbers or letters that form a unique code, which is translated from sound into light, sent through space to a satellite, and bounced back to earth where it is transmitted via more power and utility lines to the telephone of the person you are contacting—all in a few seconds' time.

Distant healing with Reiki involves the use of a series of symbols to initiate and secure a line of communication between the Reiki practitioner and the intended recipient of the healing energy. Much like calling someone on the phone, the practitioner must think of the person who is to receive the healing, and since there is no hardware to support the connection, the practitioner's thought of the person must be quite clear.

Once this is accomplished, the practitioner uses Reiki symbols in a sequence specified by his Reiki master to make the etheric connection between the practitioner and the distant-healing client strong and stable. Then the practitioner applies his hands to send healing energy, using whatever method his teacher provides. During a distant-healing treatment, the practitioner feels the energy flow through his hands with all the power and the subtlety that he does during a hands-on client treatment. The practitioner can end the treatment when he has felt a downward shift in the energy flow, signaling that the client has received sufficient Reiki to begin the work of accelerated and deep-level healing.

To continue this simple analogy, the symbols for distant healing, which are usually drawn in the air, do something rather like the number and letter buttons on your push-button phone: they send an energy signal that gets the connection going and they sustain it through the duration of your "call"—the distant-healing treatment. The Reiki distant-healing symbols, however, are a little more exotic looking than the numbers and letters on your phone.

Two of the three symbols are reminiscent of images from ancient cultures. Some designs on Minoan Bronze Age pottery and Celtic standing stones are suggestive of these symbols. One symbol is much more clearly Oriental in origin and is composed of five Japanese kanji, complex ideographs originally adopted from the Chinese language that vary in meaning according to context.

The three Reiki distant-healing symbols are traditionally regarded as sacred. They each focus the Reiki energy in particular ways to enhance the quality of healing. Because of the sacredness of the symbols, your Reiki master may ask you not to reveal them to anyone who is not also trained in Reiki to at least level II.

Although the impact of technology makes versions of the symbols readily available on the Internet, as well as in books published by teachers who are not so tradition-bound, you may not have an easy time with your conscience if you do not honor your teacher's request. At the same time, understand that the Reiki energy is dynamically alive, divinely intelligent, and evolving us all. In a year or two, your teacher may understand the importance of tradition somewhat differently and may no longer ask students to equate maintaining secrecy with understanding sacredness. If you find yourself wanting to share the symbols with another level II practitioner who did not learn them from your teacher, you may want to check back with your teacher by phone or by assisting at a level II class.

The First Symbol

The first symbol is a spiral form drawn in a specific way. This symbol evokes the beauty of a nautilus shell and the magnificent sweep of a galaxy (see figure 11.1). It echoes the visual pattern of the DNA that holds our genetic code, and the cresting of a wave that crashes on a beach tumbling what the sea holds into sand. Forms similar to it are depicted in the artifacts of ancient cultures all over the world, an acknowledgment of the geometry of power—a rendering of the mathematical symbol pi, used to denote exponential increase and growth.

A Reiki practitioner properly attuned in a level II class to the use of the distant-healing symbols uses the first symbol, or power symbol, to request an

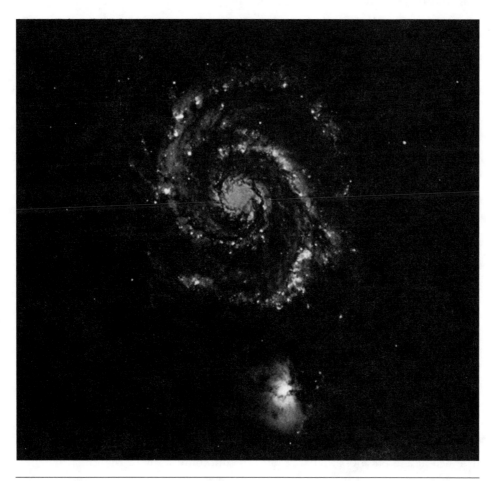

Figure 11.1. *The whirlpool galaxy in the constellation Canes Venatici reminds some practitioners of the first symbol.* UCO/Lick Observatory image.

increase in the flow of Reiki energy for the purpose of hands-on or distant healing, or to initiate a method of distant healing. For example, the practitioner might draw a large power symbol over a client laying face up on a bodywork table, extending from the base of the sternum to the pubic bone, so that all the Basic I hand positions will receive a power increase. When using this symbol, the practitioner says its Japanese name three times before, during, or after drawing it with the flat of his hand.

This symbol can also be "stacked," drawn multiple times, to call for a rapid and strong increase in Reiki power to an area of the body that has just been injured or traumatized and is in need of emergency care: a Reiki practitioner who has suffered a steam burn on her hand while cooking some vegetables might make this symbol repeatedly over the burned area to lessen pain and minimize blistering and scarring. The symbol can also be used singly or stacked in daily self-treatment to focus increased Reiki energy on a specific area of the body, for example on the Basic I hand positions, or on an extra position over an ankle that is prone to sprains.

Once the first symbol has been introduced and students have had a chance to practice writing it on paper and in the air with their hands, the Reiki master may invite them to set up treatment tables, pair up, and practice using the symbol in hands-on treatment. This gives each student the opportunity to use the symbol with some, or all, of the standard and extra hand positions used during client work. This ensures that the practitioner feels knowledgeable about the use of the symbol and is apprised of the change in the flow of energy that occurs with its use.

The Second Symbol

The second symbol is also relatively simple in form and rather primitive looking. Some Reiki masters liken this image to a bow and arrow that shoots into the heart, while others see it as the face and head of a man (see figure 11.2). These metaphors, reflecting the wide variations in how the symbol is drawn, are somewhat indicative of the different uses Takata presented for this symbol: to establish mental and emotional balance, and to communicate with the inner being.

Some of the Reiki masters taught by Takata learned to use this symbol on the body and in distant healing to work on the aura; some to work on the chakras; some to work with the client's inner being to heal unresolved feelings and unhealthy thought patterns that contributed to the development of a medical condition. All these methods serve the same end: healing the emotional and mental states that may hold a client back from complete and permanent healing. (All these methods continue to be taught by the many traditional Reiki masters who are "descended" from the original twenty-two Takata initiated, as well as those she taught who are still teaching.)

Practitioners who learn the "intuitive Reiki" method of distant healing are able to talk with Dr. Usui, Dr. Hayashi, and Mrs. Takata and to receive guidance. Unfortunately, however, only a very few of the Reiki masters taught by Takata learned this method, and most of these people teach it only to their level III students. Reverend Beth Gray, who was recognized as a gifted clairvoyant before learning Reiki, was given the method to pass along to her level II students, some of whom now, as teachers, continue instruction in this method. If you are already a level I or level II Reiki practitioner and would like to learn this method, find one of these teachers to learn specifics and to receive attunements as necessary to support the development of Reiki-guided intuitive abilities.

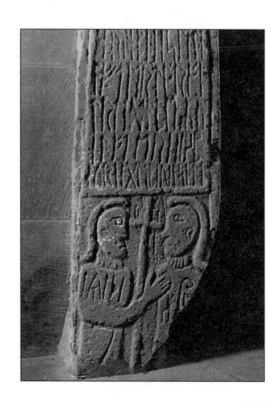

Figure 11.2. The carved figures on the Great Urswick cross-shaft are reminiscent of some versions of the second symbol. Copyright Department of Archaeology, Durham University.
Photograph: T. Middlemass.

A properly attuned level II Reiki practitioner can use the second symbol in hands-on and in distant-healing treatments to bring greater emotional and mental balance. When drawing this symbol with the flat of his hand, the practitioner uses a specific sequence of strokes and says the symbol's Japanese name three times. The second symbol may be used after the first symbol, over the client's body, to bring increased healing to the emotional and mental layers of the energy field around the body (the aura), as well as to the physical body. This symbol may also be used after completing a client treatment to balance an individual energy center (or chakra), such as the heart.

To do so, the practitioner stands at the side of the treatment table, places one hand underneath the client's back at the level of his heart, and with the other hand draws the second symbol a few inches over his heart. Then the practitioner listens to her hands for the flow of the energy to turn on, become steady, and then diminish, before moving to another position or completing the treatment.

This symbol is not normally stacked. Drawing it once is sufficient to request the Reiki energy to focus on emotional and mental healing. The symbol can also be used in hands-on self-treatment in the same ways described above to focus healing energy on feelings and thoughts that are holding stress, illness, or disease. This can be a wonderful way to help prevent a relapse of a cold or more serious condition; it can also be used effectively to gradually free a person from the negative patterns of beliefs and expectations that sometimes accompany chronic conditions, preventing complete recovery.

Once students have had an opportunity to practice drawing the second symbol, the Reiki master may send the students back to the treatment tables, in pairs, to experience using the symbol hands-on in the ways described above, or in other ways that serve the same end: restoration of emotional and mental clarity, health, and balance. Practitioners appreciate the chance to experience for themselves the subtle change in focus of the Reiki energy through the use of this symbol.

The Third Symbol

The third symbol looks Japanese, and indeed it is. Composed of five separate kanji, the complex ideographic characters in this phrase combine to create many beautiful meanings. Usually, however, this symbol is translated as, "The

God in me greets the God in you." This symbol is used to establish the connection needed for Reiki distant healing to occur.

When a Reiki practitioner uses the third symbol, the many strokes used to complete the kanji (varying from twenty to twenty-four) are drawn in a specific sequence with the flat of the hand; the practitioner says the Japanese name of the symbol three times. Although in her book *Essential Reiki,* nontraditional Reiki master Diane Stein reports using this symbol during hands-on healing to rescript past traumatic events, my research on traditional methods thus far does not describe this use. Traditional Reiki masters present the third symbol as exclusively used for distant healing. For this reason, there is no table practice; however, due to its complexity, the practice of drawing the symbol on paper may require an hour or more.

When I learned Reiki level II in 1987, students practiced drawing each of the three symbols for an hour; at the end of the class, all of the practice drawings of the symbols were collected (and later destroyed), as my teacher had promised Takata. This made memorizing the symbols perfectly while still in class extremely important. Now many traditional Reiki masters allow students to take their practice drawings home with them. Sometimes they ask that the students destroy the drawings when they feel sure of the strokes; sometimes they request that the students keep the drawings in a private file or drawer for their own reference. This seems a better solution than having the students refresh faltering memory with pictures of the symbols that are publicly available, but not necessarily the same as those taught by their Reiki master.

In a traditional Reiki class in which three attunements are given, the Reiki master will attune students to one symbol at a time, making the first, second, or third symbol the focus of each attunement. In a traditional Reiki class in which only two attunements are given, the students will be attuned to all three symbols simultaneously. These attunements are said to be of double strength because the practitioner's ability to channel the healing energy "increases by 100 percent."

Although there is a definite increase in the Reiki practitioner's ability to channel the healing energy and to do so with much greater sensitivity to the energy's myriad expressions, access to an infinite source of healing energy is just that. The actual amount of energy available to flow through a practitioner's hands does not change: all-that-is is all-that-is! What does change, however, is the practitioner's ability to consciously access the energy. This is expanded in a very important way: Now the practitioner is able to make the "hands on, Reiki on" connection that begins the flow of healing energy when the person he is treating is not physically present. He does this by thinking of the person, asking him to be present to heart and spirit through the use of the distant-healing symbols, and offering him Reiki healing for his own good and the good of all concerned. This ensures that the person receiving the energy can freely accept or reject its healing properties as he sees fit.

After learning the three distant-healing symbols, practicing the use of the first and second symbol on a client on the table, and being empowered with at least one of the level II attunements, the Reiki practitioner is likely to be sent home from the first class session with two assignments: work on yourself, incorporating the symbols as you have been taught, until you fall asleep; and practice drawing the symbols, both on paper and in the air.

At the next class session, after having a chance to collect a cup of herbal tea and find their chairs, Reiki practitioners may relate the results of their self-treatment using the symbols. While the noticeable increase in energy may surprise some of them, the gentle and beneficial effects of the Reiki will already be quite familiar, so this part of the class may be brief.

The Reiki master will usually follow this discussion with question-and-answer time, both to review the previous instruction and clarify its conceptual content. The final Reiki II attunement precedes instruction and practice of a distant-healing method.

Takata deliberately taught Reiki distant healing using many different methods, and asked those she taught to keep symbols and methods secret. During the last few years, later generations of Reiki masters and practitioners, not sworn to this vow, have begun to openly discuss such differences, and as a consequence, after much confusion, challenge, and debate, have had to relinquish any proprietary claim to the "right" method of doing Reiki.

Yet as our minds have struggled to make sense of what Takata presented, our hands have continued the work of healing. Here, with our hands on a client, we know the essential truth she wanted us to embrace: the energy itself is the true teacher and the true healer. Takata could not direct it to work in one way or another any more than we can. She simply knew, as we can now know, that it would work *always*.

200

Takata taught at least seven distinct distant-healing methods to her level II students (and to the twenty-two Reiki masters she initiated who subsequently traveled around the world teaching Reiki with all the "variety-is-the-spice-of-life" style with which they had been taught). All of the methods involve thinking of a person who is in need of healing; offering Reiki healing to be used for the highest good, with the permission of the person being sent the healing; and then using the Reiki distant-healing symbols to activate the healing energy flow. The methods can also be used to offer Reiki healing to pets, to places, to families, to organizations, and so on.

All of the methods taught by Takata work; each has advantages and disadvantages. Some of the methods direct healing energy to the whole person, so that a complete distant-healing treatment can be given quickly—often in fifteen minutes or less. These treat all levels of a person's being, including all the layers of the aura. The disadvantage of such methods is that getting accurate impressions about changes in the client's condition can be difficult. Other methods direct healing energy to the client one hand position at a time, just as if the client were on a treatment table—and can take just as long. These methods enable the practitioner to monitor changes and improvements in the client's condition very precisely.

As Reiki practitioners—and Reiki masters—gradually begin to discuss their differences in practice more openly, with love and trust in the energy as their teacher and in a spirit of friendship for others engaged in the same work, healing occurs within individuals and within communities, small, large, and as big as the world itself.

PRACTICE: SELF-TREATMENT AND CLIENT TREATMENT

Because the value of Reiki is best realized through experience, most traditional Reiki masters require their level II students to practice distant healing several times under supervision. This may mean that a student is asked to practice on himself, then on someone in the room or on someone unknown to him.

When I teach the distant-healing method I ask my students to work on themselves, then (with reference help from a picture) on someone with a medical condition unknown to them. Since a full treatment using this method takes as long as a complete hands-on self-treatment or treatment on a client, I allow an hour and a half to two hours for each of these practice sessions. Always there is a lot of discussion afterward about the method and about the meaning of any impressions received. There is also an opportunity for feedback between students who have exchanged pictures on their reports of the energy flow in response to the client's needs. The accuracy of the students' Reiki hands applied in distant healing is often quite surprising to them, even with a foundation of hands-on experience.

These practice sessions are essential to each student's understanding that her hands function just as powerfully using distant healing as they do when she treats a client in person. Also, to some extent, they eliminate the surprise of perceptions of the client's physical body: breathing, heartbeat, a pulse. When the student discovers that everyone else in the room is having these same kinds of perceptions, she is better able to get over her astonishment and to focus simply on sending healing.

This is also an opportunity to reinforce the importance of note-taking to record a client's progress during the Reiki distant-healing session, even though this means moving the hands out of the standard hand positions. Impressions of the body's energy needs are best recorded as they occur—they are often so fleeting that memory of them may be gone by the time the session is over. For those who are uncomfortable with pen and paper, a tape recorder is recommended.

The notes may be minimal and still have value, as are these notes from a distant healing I did, using myself as the client:

Basic I

9:32	Position 1: Mild warmth, tingling, more on right. Seasonal allergies starting?
9:34	Position 2: Stronger heat.
9:35	Position 3: Feel mild heat up into my face. Prickly. Hand itchy over right side.
9:40	Position 4: Strong heat, more draw on right.
9:41	Abdominal extra: Hot. Prickly, especially in lower position.
9:43	Lower T: Mild tingling.
9:45	Upper T: Heat, mild tingling.
9:46	Heart: Medium draw, heat. Prickly. Again, impression of allergies.

Basic II

9:47	Position 1: Impression allergies might be helped with increased vitamin C and pantothenic acid. More draw over left side.
9:52	Position 2: Right hand only. Left hand still in position 1.
9:55	Position 2: Left hand caught up.
9:56	Position 3: Almost no draw.
9:57	Position 4: Medium prickly draw.

Basic III

9:58	Position 1: Mild draw.
10:01	Position 2: Mild draw.
10:04	Position 3: More on left side.
10:05	Position 4: Hot over kidneys. Drink extra water.
10:07	Position 5: More on left side.
10:08	Position 6: Would like a walk today.
10:10	T: Toasty warm over coccyx.
10:12	Session concluded.

While the intuitive impressions that accompanied the hand positions in this treatment were few, they were enough to get me started on buffered vitamin C in my juice with breakfast that day, a small preparation to make for dealing with seasonal allergies. The notes also show that I am in fairly good health: none of the positions draw for very long (the result of many Reiki treatments) or are "hot," except for my kidneys (which are congenitally infection-prone). Such notes from repeated distant healings, recording the sensations and impressions received, can form a record of the practitioner's—or the client's—progress to wellness and health.

Notes can be shared with the client, but should otherwise be regarded as confidential. If the same impressions, as recorded above, had come to me while I sent distant healing to a client, I would have presented my comments verbally, reframing my impressions as suggestions, or I would have made a written copy of my notes for the client, being careful to write in clear, complete sentences and questions and to avoid any indication of diagnosis, prognosis, or prescription. For example, "allergies might be helped with increase in vitamin C and pantothenic acid," might have been rewritten: "Would you consider taking a vitamin-B complex and vitamin-C supplement in advance of allergy season? I think it might be helpful to you."

After having had an opportunity to share Reiki stories, ask questions, and do their first Reiki distant healing, students are attuned for the second and last time during the level II class. With this attunement the students are able to perceive more intuitively and to feel much more subtle sensations of energy flow through the hands. Not only are they readily able to feel the energetic connection of the distant-healing treatment, but they are also more cognizant of the energy fields around the body. They can scan the aura and the chakras—even though they may not know the layers of the aura or the location of each chakra—and find what is in balance and what is out of balance simply by listening to their hands. Where the Reiki energy draws strongly, their hands hover, sending healing to mind, heart, body, and spirit. When the energy flow becomes less intense, they know (from hands-on experience) to move their hands to another area that needs healing. This is one of the ways in which Reiki energy medicine heals all levels of being.

WORKING WITH PAST MASTERS

Although not every traditional Reiki master teaches the distant-healing method with communication (as taught by Takata to Rev. Beth Gray and a few others), I feel blessed to be able to pass on this wonderful resource to my students to assist in complete and permanent healing and to make available the guidance of Dr. Usui, Dr. Hayashi, and Hawayo Takata for any question about Reiki. For this reason, late in the class I ask the students to send distant healing, practicing the method they have just been taught, to one of these past Reiki masters. This practice is one I encourage them to do often on their own, whenever they need clear guidance and access to wisdom.

What follows is the transcription of one of my early distant-healing sessions with Takata, using the Reiki communication method she taught. The session began with a request to learn more about using Reiki for healing the aura.* It reads—and feels—much like listening and talking to her in person.

---

*In the biography of Takata presented by Larry Arnold and Sandy Nevius in *The Reiki Handbook,* they write that before learning Reiki herself, Takata wondered "how . . . these healers [were] able to tell her about pains in her body merely through touching—and sometimes even without touching—her body . . ."[1]

Takata: *"The aura is impossible to describe adequately. What human beings perceive of it in color and light is the merest suggestion of its nature. It is as complex as the physical human brain or the human body. It has subtle pathways like the neural connections in the brain and the nerve pathways in the body.*

"It is Self, and self, too—the relationship of divine to human awareness expressed in a sub-physical—no—supra-physical form. The transcendent force of the Reiki energy vitalizes and restores the aura to health, too.

"Human awareness—conscious awareness—is often quite limited, and when it is mired in sensations of physical pain, it is difficult to transmute the contracted life-force energy and refocus attention to the greater health always present, but this is what occurs when work of Reiki treatment is focused on the auric layers or levels.

"The aura is much better able to disperse and dissolve the idea of a disease process than the lymph system, say, or the spleen. But treatment on both layers—hands on the physical body and hands on the energy body—is required for easy removal of chronic symptoms; otherwise relapse can, and often does, occur. This is no fault of the practitioner directed to treat, hands-on, physical symptoms, but it is something that, having learned through your experience, you need to share.

"Just as the body stores the memory of physical trauma, accident, and disease in each affected cell as well as in the brain, so does the energy body store the memory of a thought that manifested as physical pain in its many component parts. Then the idea of disease can precipitate—or relapse can occur—again. This is why chronic illness can be difficult to treat to complete recovery.

"Knowing one layer of the aura from another does not matter. Knowing one chakra from another does not matter. These are paradigms—descriptive models of the energy-body systems. And these are but two of many.

"What matters for a Reiki practitioner is not being able to see the aura or its colors or the chakras and their colors and symbols associated with them. What matters is to be able to listen with the hands. There is no direction needed and rarely will any be taken by the Reiki energy when auric work is done, for it knows the complexity of the energy body infinitely well, and far better than humankind has so far understood. Only allow the hands to move over the energy body, feeling areas of intense heat or other activity and to pause in those places until the flow is steadied and then diminished. As you

felt last night, the energy body receives and distributes the energy of Reiki with grace and ease, and pain diminishes, because now not only the manifestation of pain but the thought of pain and the feeling of pain and the belief in pain and the attitudes that originally had drawn forth the pain are all being healed. As these heal, physical healing must quicken even more.

"*Hand positions are not important. Do a full physical treatment first, and where any physical symptom lingers, scan the area for heat and energy activity and work in that place until the energy has distributed and the pain is dispersed. That point [of pain] is a nexus of weakness in the aura. It is equivalent to working on a chakra, only a chakra is a permanent energy center. The auric overlayer of a point of pain is a temporary energy center—blocked, constricted, damaged, weakened—and in need of Reiki energy. It is a center for a practitioner's focus—like Band-Aiding.*"

Author: "*Would following up a full hands-on treatment with treatment of chakras make sense?*"

T: "*Try it sometime. It makes wonderful sense.*

"*Understand that for most physical illnesses, treatment is best hands-on, because the condition is acute. It is only when something is severe, chronic, or terminal, or relapse threatens, that auric healing becomes just as important.*"

A: "*What about working on someone who is unhappy?*"

T: "*What do you think? Work in the aura over the heart and the mind to begin, and listen to your hands for all the rest.*"

While this transcription reads like a dialogue with a teacher, many Reiki communication notes are not so easy to understand. The energy can use any of our inner senses to give us information about healing that we need to help our client or to help ourselves. This means that information may be presented to us in words—heard, as if spoken aloud, or seen, as if read—or as music, as visual images, as scents, as tastes, as tactile sensations, as feelings, and as indefinable "knowings." Learning to notice such myriad impressions, to note them without projecting emotion or interpretation, to ask for necessary clarification, and to offer them to a client in a way that will be helpful takes practice in this method of distant healing and in presentation. (If you are interested in learning more about this method, please see *Intuitive Reiki for Our Times*.)

HEALING THE WORLD WITH REIKI

As I mentioned in an earlier chapter, when I first asked my level II teacher whether Reiki distant healing could be sent to the whole world, she hesitated before giving me an answer, and then advised against it. Six months later, during another level II class at which I assisted, another student asked the same question, and she told the class that she didn't see why it couldn't be done.

Because the whole planet needs healing, I present a second distant-healing method to my students to practice during class. This method is one that I learned after I became a teacher. It is extremely efficient compared to the distant-healing method I first learned; a treatment usually takes only ten or fifteen minutes. For this reason, it is practical for many Reiki practitioners to do every day.

Here is the method:

1. Lift your hands up in front of you, at eye level or chest level, whatever is comfortable, with a few inches in between and with your palms facing each other (see figure 11.3).
2. Think of the earth between your hands. Name the whole earth or the part of the earth to which you want to send healing.
3. Offer Reiki healing.

Figure 11.3

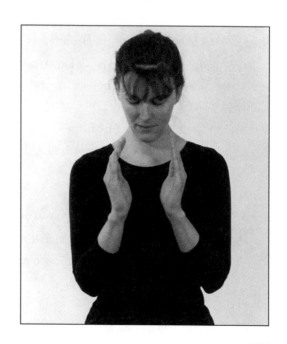

4. Acknowledge free will and higher purpose by saying something like this: "You are free to accept or reject this healing for the highest good of all concerned."

5. Make the Reiki symbols for distant healing, using whatever symbol sequence you have been taught. Then return to position the hand with which you drew the symbols.

6. Listen to the energy between your hands and allow healing.

7. When you feel the flow of energy begin to diminish, you may close the distant-healing session with an expression of thanks or a prayer of blessing, then break off the connection by blowing into the space between your hands, by clapping, or by rubbing your hands together.

This method can be adapted to focus on specific political situations; communities affected by natural disasters, famine, or disease; or environmental concerns, such as a spreading oil spill. (I usually send healing to "the biosphere of the planet earth," but sometimes students want to work on the Amazon rainforests or Alaskan coastal waters or peace in the Middle East.)

On the days that you remember to do this simple practice, the earth and all the people you encounter may seem more beautiful, more peaceful, more capable of kindness. As with all Reiki healing, this serves to heal not only the intended recipient, but the practitioner as well.

If you are not yet a level II Reiki practitioner and you would like to try sending healing energy to the world, you might experiment as follows:

1. Lift your hands up in front of you, at eye level or chest level, whatever is comfortable, with a few inches in between and with your palms facing each other.

2. Think of the earth between your hands. Name the whole earth or the part of the earth to which you want to send healing.

3. Offer a prayer for the earth's healing.

4. Imagine white light flowing into you from above, through your heart, and then through your hands.

5. Feel as deeply as you can your love for this planet that is your home and allow the energy of your love to flow through your heart, and then through your hands.

6. Allow time for healing. If you have any perception of the physical sensations that accompany energy flow, wait until they lessen in intensity or stop; or work intuitively, and let your hands stay in place for as long as it feels right.

7. Close with an expression of thanks, shake out your hands, and trust that the earth will receive the healing you have offered.

REIKI LEVEL II CERTIFICATION

Learning distant healing in a traditional Reiki level II class is exciting and joyful. Suddenly, boundaries of time and space are shown to be transparent. Because Reiki can be sent into the past, to life-scarring traumatic events, many practitioners discover that deeper healing than they have previously experienced is now possible. Because Reiki can be sent into the future, to situations that are expected to be stressful, the practitioner can become comfortable with an even more optimistic outlook. And the knowledge that healing can be sent to someone in need, who is far away, simply satisfies the heart.

Like level I, the conclusion of the level II class is marked with a ceremony, a certificate, moments of congratulation, and sometimes a photograph of smiling faces. Yet this is no real conclusion, but a continuation of the path already begun; what is being celebrated is not completion, but initiation to a new level of awareness and a deeper commitment to service and self-development through Reiki.

12

BEYOND THE REIKI II CLASS

Although the Reiki master may not see the level II students again for months or years, she may leave them with an assignment: thirty consecutive days of distant-healing practice. This is one way to ensure that the symbols, memorized in class, are not soon forgotten. (Even if the teacher has allowed the students to take notes on the symbols, the notes will not always be available; the symbols need to be known by heart and hand.)

This is also a way to make the student aware of the broader opportunities for Reiki healing that are now open to him: the cousin he has not seen since he was twelve; his retired elementary school teacher; the homeless person he passes on his walk to the bus station; his best friend, who doesn't want to talk about Reiki; his dog, who has to go to the vet for a bad cough; the accident victim reported as "hospitalized and in critical condition" on the evening news; the missing child pictured on the back of the milk carton; the cut flowers from his garden that he would like to have last all weekend; the "crisis-management" atmosphere at his job. These are a few of the countless concerns to which he can send healing with Reiki.

As he gains a foundation of experience, he may find that he experiments. Can he send distant healing in his sleep? Can he help the police find the missing child? Can he charge a cleared crystal with Reiki energy to hold healing? Can he use Reiki to help himself change a bad habit, such as smoking? Can he use Reiki to help himself realize a dream or achieve a goal?

Some traditional teachers will talk about such possibilities during a level II class, but most will focus discussion entirely on the matter of learning and practicing the distant-healing symbols, their use in hands-on Reiki, and their use in a distant-healing method. Within the usual time allotted to a level II class, this is a lot to accomplish. The teacher trusts the energy itself to continue teaching the practitioner long after the class is finished.

ASSISTING AT A LEVEL II CLASS

Just as many practitioners of hands-on healing enjoy taking advantage of the opportunity to assist at level I classes, whenever their teacher is in town, so do more advanced practitioners. This is a terrific way to recharge Reiki hands, even though reattunement may not be offered. This is also an excellent way to review the symbols and distant-healing method, to learn new uses for distant healing, and to get questions answered privately or publicly, where the answers may spark discussion and help other practitioners, too.

There is generally no charge for a return visit to a level II class; most practitioners freely give of themselves by sharing Reiki stories, helping with students' hand positions, and answering students' questions. Their presence, their hearts, and their hands, flowing with Reiki energy, help light the classroom with love. This makes assisting at a Reiki II class a happy event and an excellent opportunity for practitioners and teacher to stay in touch.

ADDING REIKI II TO A PROFESSIONAL PRACTICE

Massage therapists and bodyworkers who offer Reiki as one of their primary modalities are often curious about how to bring in the use of the distant-healing symbols to enhance their hands-on work. Usually the best way to determine this is to ask the client. If the client has specifically requested Reiki and the practitioner explains that using some newly learned advanced techniques will increase the flow of energy, the client may be quite eager to experience the effects. (If the client has not requested Reiki or indicated an openness to try this modality, do not press for permission; simply use the modalities the client prefers.)

If the client has requested Reiki and begins a session face down on the treatment table, the first symbol can be drawn over the back to increase the healing she receives in this area; when the client rolls over on the treatment table so that she is face up, relaxed, with eyes closed, the same symbol can also be used.

Most clients will be aware on some level that hand motions are being made in the air above them. If the client is familiar with the therapeutic touch method of stroking the aura, this may not raise questions. However, if the client seems at all uncomfortable, it is best to use only hands-on Reiki.

Because massage therapists and bodyworkers who offer Reiki present it as one item on a menu of modalities, there is no need to make a change on a business card, nor is there any reason to indicate attainment of level I or level II certification. Someone familiar with Reiki will appreciate the difference, but as an introduction to the community the practitioner serves, the word "Reiki" is usually sufficient.

A Reiki practitioner who has established a dedicated practice exclusively using hands-on Reiki may want to indicate training in the advanced course on a business card or a brochure. However, people may or may not be willing to pay the same fee that they pay for hands-on treatment for distant healing for themselves or others. Depending upon the amount of time that a practitioner dedicates to doing a distant healing, she might charge the same rate she charges for hands-on Reiki (comparable to standard fees in her area for massage), or reduce the rate accordingly to reflect a shorter investment of her time. At the same time, while many professional Reiki practitioners ask as much as a massage therapist for a half-hour or hour hands-on treatment, they may sometimes do distant healing at no charge, because requests for it are made casually:

> *"My sister-in-law is going to be operated on this afternoon. Do you think you could send her some healing?"*

212

"I just found out my husband slipped on the pavement on his way to work, and now he's at the hospital having his ankle looked at. Could you possibly send him some Reiki?"

While it is gracious to say, "Yes, of course, I'd be glad to," practitioners who make this a habit frequently end up with a long list of clients. If they are comfortable with the commitments they have made and are able to offer treatment to all those they have promised, they will be able to feel good about their service. If, however, they feel overburdened by the number of requests that come to them, they should consider saying, clearly but compassionately, "No, I don't think I'll be able to get to it today." They might add, "Perhaps it's time you considered learning Reiki yourself."

DECIDING TO TEACH: REIKI LEVEL III

The commitment to teaching Reiki can arise out of the simple, practical desire to increase the number of Reiki hands in the world. Sometimes a Reiki practitioner's frustration with more requests for hands-on or distant healing than she can handle translates into a sharp awareness of this need. Sometimes the Reiki practitioner has harbored a desire to teach from the moment he first heard of Reiki. Whatever the level of preparation, a practitioner considering becoming a traditional Reiki master is expected to teach Reiki, not just to treat clients with Reiki.

While some may decide that they wish to continue in their present well-established careers and to teach only one or two students at a time on an as-needed or as-requested basis, most of those who train to teach will find that Reiki becomes an important life focus. Some will work exclusively teaching Reiki classes and providing Reiki treatments, while others will teach Reiki part-time and continue to hold down jobs as computer programmers or kindergarten teachers or landscape architects—whatever work they are guided to do in the world. This can allow them to support themselves, their families, and their ongoing Reiki practice; foster their creative expressions; and ground the intensely spiritual joy of teaching Reiki with other forms of constructive community involvement.

CHOOSING A REIKI MASTER
FOR LEVEL III

Traditionally the master course in Reiki is by invitation of a Reiki master. At this point in time, however, many Reiki masters are open to being approached by any level II Reiki practitioner who feels strongly committed to continuing work with Reiki, even if the practitioner does not feel ready to commit to teaching yet. Discussing the teacher's availability and willingness to teach a master course, prerequisites, course content, and other details enables the practitioner to get a clear sense of whether or not this teacher and the program of instruction are right for him.

While the master-course content, beyond the level III attunement and instruction in how to do attunements, is up to the Reiki master, some traditional masters ask their level III students to commit to a period of instruction and apprenticeship that may require from six months to a year or more. This ensures that the student will have the opportunity to assist at several level I and II classes, assuming a gradually more active role, and also gives the Reiki master a chance to observe the student's first classes, observing quietly and commenting afterward on the student's presentation.

Practitioners with very little experience, as well as those who have worked with Reiki for years, approach Reiki masters about level III training. Traditionally what is required is experience and the commitment to teach Reiki. My Takata-trained teacher asked that anyone who wanted to learn level III from her have at least five years of professional practice in which Reiki was the only modality offered before approaching her with this request.

My own requirements are less stringent: although I require prospective Reiki master students to be experienced Reiki practitioners with a deep commitment to personal healing and spiritual growth, I am willing to discuss the process of training and certification even with those who are relatively new to Reiki. I prefer to teach the master course to practitioners who have dedicated hundreds of hours to hands-on and distant healing and who have assisted at both level I and II classes. However, sometimes I am guided to accept students who have less experience but a very high level of motivation. I believe that strict requirements deter only those whose commitment is not deep and sincere. I am not interested in having as a student anyone who wants instant gratification, a lucrative career change overnight, or to "try out" teaching Reiki.

Less traditional teachers make Reiki level III instruction into a weekend seminar offering. While I understand that temptation to take such a course may be strong, and those who choose to do so may do so with the best intentions, I feel no inclination to "whip up" a two-day course syllabus so that I can take advantage of this trend. I know that Reiki is with me for life. I also know that every experience I have of this Reiki energy is uplifting, and I realize that the process of teaching involves not only the transmission of conceptual knowledge but also an energetic exchange. While these are effectively accomplished during the two or three days of level I and II classes, the level III attunement is initiation into a much deeper sensitivity to the energy and appreciation of its healing effects. It is during the course of the apprenticeship that the energy "visits" in an extraordinarily intense and loving way on every occasion when teacher and students meet for practice and discussion. This is what I want my level III students to experience: the energy's presence. In this way they will be transformed into Reiki masters who are, indeed, still students of the energy, still learning their own lessons all the time, but who are able to teach what they know because they feel the Reiki energy's presence and know that the energy is the true teacher.

Appendix 1

HAWAYO TAKATA'S STORY OF MIKAO USUI

Why did Hawayo Takata turn Mikao Usui's quest for enlightenment into a search for Christ's method of performing healing miracles? Why did she describe him as a teacher at a Christian school for boys and even, at times, as a professor at Doshisha University? Why did she include an episode in the journey of his life that took him to the University of Chicago, among its scholars of religion? Hiroshi Doi has found no evidence of Usui's employment at Doshisha University, nor of his attendance at the University of Chicago.

Perhaps we will never truly know or fully understand Takata's reasons. Although it is possible that she simply wanted to make the story of Mikao Usui's life more appealing to her listeners, it seems more likely that she took very seriously Dr. Hayashi's instruction to her to safeguard Reiki through World War II and its aftermath. As someone of Japanese descent, born on the island of Hawaii, she must have been acutely aware of the anti-Japanese sentiment in this country during that time period and perhaps experienced its cruel expression herself. After the war, many Americans still felt a residue of anger and resentment against those of Japanese, German, and Italian descent. This fear of foreigners was exacerbated in the 1950s by the blacklisting of suspected Communists, the espionage trial and conviction of the Rosenbergs, and the Cold War.

We now live in a world which is far less tolerant of racial and ethnic discrimination, but that doesn't mean we should forget that its divisiveness shaped the lives of countless millions of people in the last century, forcing many of them to make hard choices that might now seem unimaginable to us. Let us remember that Hawayo Takata demonstrated again and again the ability to listen to that inner voice that guided her first to Japan and to Dr. Hayashi's Reiki clinic. Let us allow for the possibility that she remained guided in her teaching of Reiki throughout her life. Let's appreciate her story of Mikao Usui's life as a parable-like tale, which demonstrates one man's dedication and wisdom—and be inspired by the life-lessons it presents. How can we not feel grateful to the storyteller who carefully crafted this tale in such a way that the truth of Reiki would survive "the infamy" of World War II, and she would be allowed to continue to practice and teach Reiki through the next four decades?

Did Hawayo Takata know the "true" story? I think she did. When Tom Rigler first trained me in the Usui Reiki Ryoho (traditional Japanese) techniques in 2001, my memory was jarred by some of the information he shared about Mikao Usui's early employment, which was quite varied. In addition to working as a journalist, Usui had worked as a secretary and as a prison warden. Where and when had I heard this information before? I shrugged off the feeling of familiarity and convinced myself that I must simply have accepted the "new" material because I had gone over it so many times in my mind. Then, during the writing of this revised edition, I woke from an early morning dream: I was assisting in one of Rev. Beth Gray's classes, standing in the back of the familiar conference room at the hotel in Flemington, New Jersey, where I had, in fact, assisted at Reiki I and II classes so many times. She had been challenged by a student who wanted to know what had prompted Mikao Usui to seek enlightenment.

In response, my teacher told a different story than the one we had come to expect: Mikao Usui had pursued many occupations. He had worked as a newspaper journalist. He had worked as a secretary to a government official. He had served as an attaché, an administrative assistant, to some naval officers. He had worked as a prison warden. He had gone into business, but had not been successful. What was the right work for him? What was the purpose of this life? In hope of finding an answer, he sought out a sage. The sage's advice to him was this: If you want to experience enlightenment, meditate until you experience it—or die. This prompted Mikao Usui to perform the twenty-one-day meditation, fast, and prayer vigil on Mount Kurama, which transformed him into a healer and spiritual teacher.

When I woke from the dream, I realized that it had been so vivid that it felt more like memory. Had I heard Beth give this answer to a student in a Reiki II class and simply repressed the memory because it did not "match" the story of Mikao Usui's life she had told in my Reiki I class and in so many at which I assisted? There was one way to find out: I phoned John Morrow, a Reiki master friend who, like me, had assisted at more than a dozen classes in the span of a few years. In fact, he had learned Reiki before me, and so had been assisting for an even longer period of time. Could he remember Beth telling this story?

"Yes, I do," he said, "and more than once." This was reassuring. "She did say that Dr. Usui had been a prison warden. That's something that's hard to forget—and yes, he pursued enlightenment because he wanted to find out the purpose of his life."[1]

However, further confirmation for the story came from an unexpected source: In *Light on the Origins of Reiki: A Handbook for Practicing the Original Reiki of Usui and Hayashi,* Tadao Yamaguchi remembers his mother telling him a very similar story. After working in a number of occupations, including as "a religious missionary and a counselor working to rehabilitate prisoners," and gaining a broad perspective on the world, Mikao Usui came to ask himself the ultimate question, "What is the true purpose of life?"[2]

It seems likely that Takata did share at least some other details of her original training with some of her Reiki master students. Copies of pages from her diary have been shared across generations of teachers, revealing that she learned techniques taught within the Usui Reiki Ryoho Gakkai and used the Japanese terms to refer to them. She also gave papers written in Japanese to some of her students. For example, John Gray has recently had translated a Japanese document that proved to be Hayashi's teaching manual (see *Hand to Hand*[3]). Beth Gray also had in her possession documents written in Japanese calligraphy, given to her by Takata. A single tantalizing photo has been published on the Internet, which shows Takata performing a Reiki treatment in Japan, surrounded by Japanese men. The caption above the image reads "Reiki Ryoho Gakkai 1937."[4]

Takata taught Reiki as Dr. Hayashi taught it to her, making some changes in order to communicate with an English-speaking audience. We might not use the term *hibiki* to describe the sensations of the Reiki energy flowing in our hands, but if we are trained in Usui Shiki Reiki Ryoho, we learn to listen to our hands. We may not be told that we are receiving *reiju,* but we are attuned repeatedly, just as students are within the Usui Reiki Ryoho Gakkai. We may be told Takata's story of Mikao Usui's life in Reiki I class and invited to see his interest in healing within a Christian context—or not—but we will learn of his awakening on Mount Kurama and understand that it was the turning point in his life, just as it was described within the Usui Memorial and just as it is still described to traditional Japanese practitioners.

And so here is Hawayo Takata's story of Mikao Usui, as told to me by Takata-trained Reiki Master Rev. Beth Gray:

Dr. Mikao Usui taught at a Christian seminary school in Kyoto in the late 1800s. One day one of his graduating students approached him with a question. The student said, "Dr. Usui, you have taught us the stories of the Bible. You have taught us the precepts of Christianity. You have prepared us to go out into the world and preach. Yet you have never taught us how to heal the lame or cure the blind as Christ did. Why is this? Can you show us the passage in the Bible where we may learn this?"

Dr. Usui answered, "I cannot teach you how to heal the sick, for I do not know how to do so myself. I do know the Bible, but I do not know any passage in the Bible which describes how Christ healed. However, your question is a good question, and it deserves an answer. I will do some research on this matter, and I will find the answer for you."

Dr. Usui began his search in the library of the Christian seminary school where he taught. He spent many hours poring over all the volumes that he thought might be in any way useful in answering his student's question, "How did Christ heal?" Finally, after days of sitting in the hard library chairs and reading until his eyes burned, he accepted the question as his own question. He determined that he would have to broaden his search to find the answer.

Dr. Usui talked to another teacher at the Christian seminary school in Kyoto about his student's request and his own frustration in finding the scholarly resources he needed to provide an answer. His friend suggested that he go to America, since Christianity had come to Japan from America, and do his research in the scholarly libraries there. Dr. Usui thought this was an excellent idea. He applied for a visa to come to America; after several months of waiting, his visa was approved. Leaving Kyoto for Chicago, Dr. Usui was full of excitement and hope that he would find the answer to his question while in America.

In Chicago, Dr. Usui studied with world-renowned scholars of religion at the University of Chicago for several years and learned much; he spent hundreds of hours in the religion section of the library, reading books about the practice of the early Christian religion, and again, he learned much. Still, he did not come across the answer to the question he was seeking. So he decided to write to as many priests, ministers, and rabbis of congregations all over America as he could, hoping that one of them might be able to answer the question of how Christ healed. Unfortunately, those who answered could only assure Dr. Usui that their work was healing the spirit; healing the body was not something that they knew anything about at all.

Dr. Usui confessed his discouragement to a friend he had made at the university. His friend had a curious answer. "Buddhism is much older than Christianity," he said. "Perhaps the practice of healing has been taught at some point in the Buddhist tradition. If so, you may be able to find out by inquiring at the Buddhist temples in your own country."

Dr. Usui gave careful consideration to this thought. He had spent years searching for the answer to his question in America, using the best scholarly resources on Christianity in the world. Although he had learned much, he had not found the answer he was seeking. His efforts had been without result; there was no more for him to do here. It was time to go home to his own country.

So Dr. Usui returned to Kyoto and set about his quest with renewed vigor. There were seventeen Buddhist temples in Kyoto. One by one he visited them all, and asked the monks who greeted him the same question: "Do you teach how to heal the way that Christ healed and the way the Buddha healed?" One by one, over and over again, the monks told him no. Finally, at the seventeenth temple he visited, the monk he talked to gave him a slightly different answer: "No, we do not teach how to heal anymore."

"What do you mean?" Dr. Usui wanted to know. "You say that you don't teach healing anymore. Are you saying that at one time you *did* teach healing?"

"Indeed, we did," the monk said. "But we do not anymore. We have lost the knowledge of healing."

Now many years had gone by since Dr. Usui had begun his studies. Although friends he had made along the way had often encouraged him, they had never been able to offer him hope of finding an answer. Now here was one small hope.

"Perhaps the healing that was once possible may be so again," Dr. Usui said, barely containing his excitement. "May I enter this monastery? May I study the books and scrolls that are in your library?"

"You are welcome," the monk assured him. "You may stay with us and study for as long as you like."

Dr. Usui immediately moved into the monastery and began to live as the Buddhist monks lived, spending much of the time that he was not in the library in meditation, fasting, and prayer. Years went by. He read all the books and scrolls that he was able to read in Japanese and in English, but he could not read the scrolls written in Sanskrit. Finally he decided that he must learn Sanskrit to complete his research. So he did.

Dr. Usui was often left to himself as he studied and began to understand individual words and then phrases and then sentences. Little by little, the parchment scrolls began to yield their secrets to him. Much that he read had been translated into Japanese or even into English, and so was already familiar to him. But one day he found a scroll that described a process of healing that was unlike anything he had read about so far. Here, written in Sanskrit, in fading ink on fragile parchment, were rituals described for calling on God—the universal life force—to direct healing energy through human hands. The rituals used symbols—beautiful, simple, primitive symbols that might have been painted by ancient man or woman on a cave wall, and elegant, complex, and more modern symbols, clearly derived from Chinese and Japanese, perhaps recorded by one of the last of the Buddhist monks in the sect to learn this traditional method of healing from a master.

Dr. Usui realized the import of what he had found: This was the method of healing Christ had used to cure the blind and to heal the sick; this was the same method the Buddha had used to perform healing; perhaps even other spiritual masters, whose names were not recorded by the people among whom they dwelt, had used this method as well. This was a sacred teaching, of great importance and great value to the world and to the individuals who learned and practiced it. Should it be returned to the "civilized" world, which, more and more, seemed to be forgetting spiritual values? Perhaps the sacred teaching had been forgotten because the world had become undeserving, and the record of the teaching should be left to fade into obscurity and the parchment to crumble into dust on the monastery shelves. Yet if, as Dr. Usui believed as a Christian, "there is a time to every purpose under heaven," Dr. Usui might have discovered this lost scroll and lost teaching because the time had come for the world to have healing. Dr. Usui felt that he could not make this decision alone.

He turned to the abbot of the monastery for guidance. He told the abbot that he had found a scroll written in Sanskrit that revealed the method of healing used by Christ and by the Buddha to heal the sick. The abbot was glad of the discovery, but like Dr. Usui, felt that the decision to reveal such a teaching to the world should be made only with the guidance of God. So it was decided that both men would meditate and fast and pray through the night and speak again in the morning.

With the sunrise, they met. The abbot told Dr. Usui to make a pilgrimage to the sacred mountain, Mount Kurama, to meditate and fast and pray for twenty-one days, and to ask God for a vision. Only if a vision came to Dr. Usui should he feel certain that he should reveal this method of healing to the world.

Dr. Usui set off for the mountain that very morning. As he left the monastery, he told a young boy who lived there, "I go to Mount Kurama to meditate and fast and pray for twenty-one days. If I do not return by the night of the twenty-first day, send someone for my bones, for surely I will be dead." The boy nodded in agreement. With that Dr. Usui began his long walk out of town, onto more and more isolated roads, then off the roads onto the mountain trails, higher and higher, until finally, wearily, he reached the mountaintop.

There he gathered twenty-one stones. He set these in a pile beside him. He sat down on the hard, cold ground and began his meditation and fasting and prayer. Day after day he sat unmoving, except to reach for a stone from the pile beside him to shift it to another pile. In this way he numbered the days as they passed. Finally, he had only a few stones left. Weak from hunger and stiff from sitting in one position, even the small stones seemed heavy to him. He doubted that he would have a vision. He thought that surely he would die.

Finally, before dawn on the twenty-first day, he reached for the last stone, his hand trembling with the effort. There had been no vision. He wondered if he would be able to make the return journey home. He tried to focus his eyes on the horizon, and just as he did so, the sun began to rise. The first ray of sunlight struck him like golden lightning. So powerful was this ray that he fell back and lay still, his eyes closed against the power of the light. Yet even with his eyes closed, he could still see this light.

Too weak to move and powerless to block the light, he surrendered to it, and he had his vision. He began to see that the intense bright light flowing into him was made of hundreds and hundreds of bubbles of light, like a river is made of droplets of rain. Each of these bubbles was one of the colors of the rainbow and glowed with iridescence. As the bubbles streamed into him, he saw that within each bubble was writing, and the writing was the same as he had read on the Sanskrit scroll. Indeed, he saw the symbols of Reiki. As he understood what he saw, the bubbles glowed golden again, and then white, and then they burst open, dissolving their energy into him. Again and again the bubbles flowed into him until finally, gently, the flow diminished and then ceased.

Dr. Usui opened his eyes to the bright golden sun of midday. He sprang up off the ground, full of happiness and strength. He had been blessed with a vision, and he felt well and strong. This is the first miracle attributed to Reiki—that he felt well and not weakened by twenty-one days of fasting and meditation.

So eager was he to share the news of his vision and to begin the work of bringing this ancient method of healing into the world that he began to run down the mountain. This was not wise on the rocky terrain of the mountaintop. He ran only a few steps when he stubbed his toe, ripping off some of his toenail and causing his toe to bleed. Naturally, he did what anyone does in this situation—he grabbed his toe. Soon he noticed that the pain was subsiding. Then there was no pain at all. He lifted up his hands. The bleeding had stopped; the toe was completely healed. This is the second miracle attributed to Reiki.

Dr. Usui proceeded down the mountain again, this time at a more rea-
sonable pace. After some time he became aware that he was hungry. He
determined that he would stop for food. When he saw a little bench with a
red cloth on it along his trail, he sat down to wait, for in Japan this is a sign
to travelers that hospitality and a meal are offered by those who live nearby.
Soon a little girl came to him where he sat on the bench and asked if he was
hungry. She was a pretty little child, but her face was swollen and distorted
and wrapped in a cloth.

Dr. Usui said, "Yes, I would be happy for some food, child, but first, I
cannot help noticing that you have wrapped your head in a cloth as if to
keep your face warm and a poultice against it. Are you all right?"

"I have a toothache. Kyoto is far down the mountain, and my father and I
cannot afford a dentist."

"May I see where it hurts? May I touch the place?"

The girl pointed to the area of her pain. Dr. Usui very gently put his palm
there.

After a moment the little girl said, "Your hand is very warm, sir." She
closed her eyes, enjoying the sensation of gentle, radiant heat. Then she
opened them again in surprise. "The pain is gone!"

Dr. Usui smiled at her and slowly lowered his hand.

She was excited. "Oh, my toothache is cured. I must tell my father. Come
with me, good monk. Come!"

The cure of the little girl's toothache is the third miracle attributed to Reiki,
and the fourth miracle is that when Dr. Usui sat down to eat a meal with these
people, and he was served hot, spicy, pickled foods, his hunger was satisfied.
He still felt strong. His fast of twenty-one days had no debilitating effect.

Dr. Usui said good-bye to the child and her father and continued his long
walk down the mountain to Kyoto. He felt in radiant health. Now he began
to consider how he should bring this healing energy to all the people. Should
he wander and trust that his footsteps would be guided on the path to those
who needed the healing energy the most? Or should he settle in one place, so
that these same people could find him?

When he finally came to the temple monastery, he was eager to talk to the
abbot, to tell him of his vision and ask for his guidance. He saw the little

boy who lived at the monastery on his way in. He told the boy that there was no need to send anyone for his bones, for he was quite well. The boy went running ahead to relay the news. A monk came out of the monastery to welcome him. Dr. Usui thanked him for his welcome and asked if he might see the abbot. This monk told Dr. Usui that the abbot was sadly indisposed, sitting with his feet in a tub, soaking them to ease crippling arthritis.

"Take me to him, please," Dr. Usui asked. The monk led him to a little room in the back of the monastery, and left Dr. Usui with the abbot. Dr. Usui bowed in greeting. Then he sat beside the abbot, asked permission to hold the abbot's aching feet in his hands, and talked. The healing energy slowly, gently, worked its miracle while Dr. Usui and the abbot talked. For hours they talked, reflecting on the responsibility of being entrusted with a vision. Finally the abbot thanked Dr. Usui for bringing him healing; he suggested that they both spend the night in prayer and meditation and fasting, and meet again in the morning to continue their talk.

They did this, and when they met again in the morning, they decided that Dr. Usui would begin to bring healing Reiki energy into the world in one corner of Kyoto that appeared to need great healing: the Beggar City.* The Beggar City is like an area of New York City run by the Mafia. Everyone who works in the Beggar City must pay the Beggar King for "protection." Dr. Usui, setting off from the monastery, was not quite sure what he was getting into.

Almost as soon as he entered the Beggar City, he was accosted by two beggars. "Give us your money," one said. "Give us your clothes," the other said.

"I have no money to give you, and I have no clothes besides these I wear on my back. I have nothing for you."

The beggars scowled at him angrily, and one lunged toward him.

"But I do have a gift for the Beggar King," Dr. Usui said.

---

*The historical details made accessible to readers through Petter's *Reiki Fire* place Dr. Usui in Tokyo treating people with Reiki immediately after his pilgrimage and meditation on Mount Kurama. However, this mountain is actually near Kyoto, the ancient capital, a city with many temples and holy places. While it may never be possible to verify all the details of this widely told story of Dr. Usui, more open exchange of information with Usui Reiki masters teaching in Japan offers the hope of knowing Dr. Usui better and appreciating his extraordinary compassion and commitment to healing more fully.

The location of Mount Kurama on the outskirts of Kyoto was confirmed in a telephone conversation with a representative of the Japanese Embassy, Washington, D.C., on November 28, 1997.

The beggar who threatened him paused. "What gift?"

"Give it to us," the other beggar said.

"No, I cannot. This gift I can give only to the Beggar King. I think he will appreciate it and perhaps give you a reward for bringing me to him."

The two beggars conferred. Finally they decided to bring Dr. Usui to the Beggar King. They blindfolded him and led him through dark, stinking alleys in the Beggar City, until, at last, they stood him before the Beggar King and removed his blindfold.

"I understand that you have something for me," the Beggar King said.

"I bring a gift for you and for all the beggars: the power of healing."

"What?!? This is not the kind of gift I was expecting. What good is it to me or to the beggars?"

"It is a gift to feel well and strong."

The Beggar King considered this. He had not gotten to be the Beggar King without being healthy, as well as crafty. "I have no use for it myself. The beggars might like it, though. You can work in the Beggar City under my protection."

"Thank you," Dr. Usui said.

"But you cannot wear those clothes," the Beggar King said. "They are much too fine. You must dress like a beggar if you are to live among the beggars."

Dr. Usui nodded in acceptance. "I will dress as a beggar, but I will not beg for food. My work is to bring healing. Will you feed me?"

The Beggar King put a hand on his chin and pondered. "You may have scraps from my table. That should sustain you."

Dr. Usui nodded again. "Then let me begin my work."

And so Dr. Usui began to give Reiki treatments to the beggars. Day after day, he walked among them and offered healing wherever he saw hurt. All the beggars he touched felt the healing power of the energy. Soon, they came to him to ask for healing. The days became weeks, and the weeks became years. The beggars became well, and some of them left the Beggar City, but still there were always new beggars coming to live there.

One day a beggar whose face seemed somehow familiar came to Dr. Usui. "Don't I know you?" he asked the beggar, and placed his hands over the man's dirty rags.

"Oh yes, Dr. Usui. You do know me. I was one of the very first beggars you healed here."

Dr. Usui was confounded. "Why are you here for healing again?" he asked. "My intention was that you reclaim your health and you go away from the Beggar City and make a new life for yourself. Didn't you do that?"

"Well, I did," the beggar admitted. "But it is hard to work all day for a living and come home tired at night and cook and then, the next day, begin all over again." The beggar shook his head. "I decided it wasn't for me. It is much easier to be a beggar."

Dr. Usui lifted up his hands and stepped away from the beggar. He was disappointed and upset. "Never again will I offer this healing energy for free. Anyone who receives it must value it. This is the last that I work in the Beggar City."

With that Dr. Usui walked away from the astonished beggar, and from all the beggars who stood open-mouthed with surprise in his wake. He left the Beggar City never to return. He went into the heart of downtown Kyoto and stood at a street corner with a torch brightly lit and held high, silhouetted against the blue sky and the midday sun. He shouted at the crowd of lunchtime passersby: "Anyone who wants to be healed and made well, and who will pay to be healed and made well, come to me. I offer healing to anyone who will value it." Although he seemed like a crazy man with his flaming torch held high to touch the sun, people heard his message and came to him. Many, many people came to him and they received healing, and they were glad to pay him for his work, for they valued it and were grateful to be able to live out their lives in the fullness of good health.

As a result of Mikao Usui's encounter with the ungrateful beggar, he adopted a set of five statements as guidelines for daily living and meditation. These statements, known as the Reiki principles or ideals, encourage us to make wise, healthy choices:

> *Just for today, do not anger.*
> *Just for today, do not worry.*
> *Be grateful. Count your blessings.*
> *Do an honest day's work.*
> *Be kind to all living things.*

Appendix 2

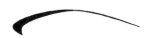

EXPLORATIONS: BOUNDLESS REIKI, BOUNDLESS LEARNING

The work and teachings of Mikao Usui, Chujiro Hayashi, and Hawayo Takata have forever changed the consciousness of this world. No longer are miracles of healing so rare. No longer does anyone need to feel powerless to do anything but pray as they sit beside the bedside of someone they love who is ill or dying. Nor does death itself need to be experienced as having the same sting. The boundary that seemed to forever separate us from the knowledge of Spirit has been dissolving.

Now, many years after Mikao Usui stepped onto the trail up Mount Kurama, more and more people find themselves on this path, and in the congenial company of others who value their own spiritual natures, their shared humanity, the other creatures who keep us company, and the earth, our shared home. What brings us together and holds us here is the universal life-force itself. Feeling the flow of this energy, experiencing it, and expressing it, we move forward. And as we move forward, and we acknowledge the presence and the power of this energy in our companions, we join hands.

What follows is an attempt to acknowledge some of these companions-in-

Spirit for their individuality, their commonality, and their inspired contributions to the practice of traditional Reiki. The descriptions of the healing methods that follow are not always based on personal experience, but on research, personal correspondence, or discussion. Because of this, no recommendations or endorsements of any of these methods can be made beyond this acknowledgment. However, because all of the methods described below are strongly based in historically accepted practice, they may safely be explored by anyone interested in deepening his understanding of Reiki.

What distinguishes traditional Reiki from non-traditional? Traditional Reiki masters offer their students repeated attunements—or reiju—to support the students' transformation into clear, conscious channels of Reiki energy. Although we all possess the natural ability to bring comfort and some healing through our hands, each attunement we receive enhances that ability, so that the channel for healing energy is opened "wider," stabilized, reinforced, and sealed for life—and each attunement we receive makes it easier for us to perceive the subtle flow and shifts of the Reiki energy through our hands. Although students are told that daily practice will certainly enhance the ability to perceive this subtle flow, most students are able to feel the transformation in their hands before the Reiki I class ends.

In traditionally taught classes in the West, Reiki I students are given four attunements; Reiki II students are given two or three attunements; and Reiki III (master) students are usually given one additional attunement. In the Usui Reiki Ryoho Gakkai in Japan, students are initiated with a single reiju or attunement, but then receive an additional attunement at every monthly meeting they attend, so that their sensitivity to the energy continually increases and their understanding of their experiences with Reiki deepens.

Traditional Reiki, both Western and Japanese, also emphasizes the importance of learning to "listen" to the flow of healing energy in the hands. In a Reiki I class, the Reiki master will often support students in accomplishing this goal by describing the many sensations that may accompany the energy's flow, as well as instructing the students in how to perceive a cycle of energy, from its onset and increase to a level intensity to its subsiding. This instruction is *always* followed by the opportunity to practice not only hand placements but this enhanced perception of subtle energy. In Japan, within the Usui Reiki

Ryoho Gakkai, the equivalent instruction is offered to Shoden level students, as they demonstrate increasing awareness of the flow of healing energy. First, they are taught that *hibiki* or "resonance" in their hands, over an area of the body, is indicative of a need for healing; then they are taught Byosen-ho, or scanning, and ultimately, Reiji-ho, or intuitive hand placement.

Because of the repetition of attunements and the emphasis on learning to listen to the hands, traditionally taught Reiki classes provide an excellent foundation for effective Reiki practice and pathwork. Such classes are well worth seeking out—and many practitioners have traveled across state lines, country borders, and continents to attend them; they are also worth waiting for—do not be disheartened to learn that you must wait a few weeks or even months to attend a traditionally taught Reiki class.

Be aware that many traditional Reiki masters in the West who trace their lineage back through Hawayo Takata and Chujiro Hayashi to Mikao Usui describe themselves as teaching "Usui Shiki Ryoho," but others, even though they teach in a traditional manner, have dropped or changed the name. John Gray, one of the earliest Reiki masters trained by Hawayo Takata, originally taught Usui Shiki Reiki Ryoho, but now teaches the Usui-Gray Integrated Reiki System. Australian native Barbara McGregor who was initiated as a Reiki master by my teacher, Rev. Beth Gray, teaches Usui Reiki. So if you are determined to find a traditionally taught class, ask your prospective teacher some key questions: How many attunements will this class include? How will I learn to sense the flow of healing energy in my hands? Will I be given the opportunity to practice doing a complete Reiki treatment?

For those who are attracted to any of the hundreds of modern variations of Reiki, you might wish to investigate classes offered through the International Center for Reiki Training (ICRT) (www.reiki.org). This organization has offered standardized classes providing one attunement at each level since 1990, performed by teachers who are required to maintain their qualifications through continuing education and a recertification process. The information presented in the classes reflects the training, interests, and dedication to research of the organization's founder William Rand: "The style we teach is a combination of the Usui/Hayashi method as taught by Mrs. Takata combined with a style based on Tibetan shamanism called Raku Kai. In 1998, after reviewing the research done in Japan, we added the [historical] Japanese Reiki techniques to our train-ing."[1] As a consequence, this style, although it departs from traditional Usui Shiki Reiki teaching in some ways, subtracting and adding some elements, still has much in common with it. The ICRT is extremely well organized and profes-sional in its presentation, and it has done much to popularize Reiki around the world. It reaches prospective students and practitioners through an extensive website, a free online newsletter, and the *Reiki News Magazine,* a glossy four-color quarterly that can be found on the stands of Borders, Barnes & Noble, and some independent bookstores. The magazine has an international circula-tion, offers many interesting articles and Reiki stories, and is committed to "honoring all lineages and schools."

If you are still tempted to learn some newly minted brand of Reiki, here are some words of caution: ask your instructor to provide a detailed description of qualifications (especially training and years of experience, both as a practitio-ner and as a teacher); ask what material the class will cover; and ask how this form of Reiki is different from traditional Reiki. If the instructor makes wildly enthusiastic claims that this form is faster, better, stronger, or more powerful, don't sign up on the spot. Ask for time to think over your decision about the class—and take that time. Be prepared to evaluate carefully the reasons given to you for changes from a traditionally taught Reiki class; recognize that ego is rarely the best teacher; and let yourself be guided by your inner wisdom before deciding how and when to go forward on your Reiki path.

GENDAI OR "MODERN" REIKI

Hiroshi Doi, author of *Iyashino Gendai Reiki-ho* or "Modern Reiki Method for Healing" and a member of the Usui Reiki Ryoho Gakkai, first established the Gendai Reiki Kyokai in Japan in 1995 for the purpose of providing instruc-tion "for modern people to use Reiki practically."[2] Doi's teachers include both a Radiance Technique Reiki master who visited Japan and Kimiko Koyama (now deceased), the sixth chairperson of the Usui Reiki Ryoho Gakkai. Drawing on the two rich traditions of Western style and Japanese Reiki, he has developed a very comprehensive instructional method that is presented in four levels: 1) "opening Reiki channel"; 2) "enhancing Reiki Power and extending the use of

Reiki"; 3) "reaching higher level of vibration of consciousness and being more creative"; and 4) "becoming a Reiki teacher."[3]

One of his missions is to set the historical record straight regarding the life of Mikao Usui and the early practice of Reiki. He, too, provides translations of key documents in Reiki history: the Gainen, portions of the Hikkei and selected poems from the Meiji Emporer, and the Usui Memorial. He asks Western Reiki masters who wish to learn Gendai Reiki to first take a workshop to establish familiarity with the techniques that have been practiced for the last eighty years in Japan. Once certified in these historical techniques, they are welcome to take the Gendai Reiki Workshop and become qualified to teach it at all levels.

For information regarding Doi's Gendai classes in North America, please contact Elyssa Matthews at kokoro@dsl.ca. Tom Rigler, one of those who sponsored Doi's first trip to the West in 1999, also travels worldwide teaching Usui Reiki Ryoho and Gendai Reiki. To contact Tom, e-mail him at lotusheart@lotusheart.us. You may also discover other Reiki masters who have trained with Doi or Rigler by keying into a search engine the words "Gendai Reiki" and the name of your state.

JIKIDEN REIKI

Tadao Yamaguchi is the son of Chiyoko Iwamoto Yamaguchi, who learned First and Second Degree Reiki directly from Dr. Chujiro Hayashi in 1938, when she was just seventeen years old, with the encouragement of her family. Her uncle, Wasaburo Sugano, had attended a Reiki training session presented by Dr. Hayashi in Osaka in 1928, and he subsequently used Reiki to cure his wife and later his elder brother of tuberculosis, a disease then considered incurable. This motivated him to continue his training with Hayashi, who acknowledged Sugano as a Shihan, or teacher, in about 1933. Chiyoko Iwamoto received her instruction in reiju (the attunement or empowerment process) from Sugano in about 1940, with Dr. Hayashi's approval.

In 1942, Chiyoko married Shosuke Yamaguchi and traveled to Manchuria, where her husband had established a business. They soon started a family, giving her the opportunity to use Reiki on her young children; eventually, she also used Reiki to help save her husband's life, after he sustained serious injuries serving Japan during the war. Tadao Yamaguchi received his first reiju when he was just five years old, so Reiki has always been an important part of his life.

In the late 1990s, Mrs. Yamaguchi made the decision to hold weekly meetings to teach Reiki to the Shihan level to her son and anyone else interested. Every Monday afternoon for over a year, she met with a small group of students, chanted the Gainen, and performed reiju. Only Tadao Yamaguchi and Rev. Hyakuten Inamoto completed this training.[4] (For more about Rev. Inamoto's Reiki classes, see "Komyo Reiki" below.)

Tadao Yamaguchi and his mother established the Jikiden Reiki Kenkyukai in 1999 to teach Reiki as Hayashi had taught it. Although Mrs. Yamaguchi made her transition from this life in 2003, Tadao Yamaguchi continues to teach Jikiden Reiki actively today. He says in his book *Light on the Origins of Reiki: A Handbook for Practicing the Original Reiki of Usui and Hayashi* (first published in Japan in 2003 and first published in an English edition in 2007): "You might be wondering what 'Jikiden' means. 'Jikiden' is a general term for the Japanese . . . that means 'directly transmitted or passed down from one's teacher' and for us the teacher is Hayashi Sensei. I named my institute and seminar 'Jikiden Reiki' because I have been trying to replicate as closely as possible the teachings passed down to my mother directly by Hayashi Sensei. . . . I have resolved to do my best."[5]

For more information on Jikiden Reiki and to learn when Tadao Yamaguchi will be teaching Jikiden Reiki at a location near you, please visit his website, www.jikiden-reiki.com.

KOMYO REIKI

Rev. Hyakuten Inamoto, a Pure Land Buddhist priest and Reiki teacher, first studied Reiki with Chiyoko Yamaguchi in weekly meetings that took place over the course of a year and that always included recitation of the Gokai (the five core statements that are known throughout the world as the Reiki principles), reiju, and practice. Because of his vow of compassionate service, he was eager to learn and grateful for the experience of the Reiki energy. His studies continued with Hiroshi Doi, who familiarized him with the techniques historically practiced within the Gakkai and who initiated him into

233

Gendai Reiki, Doi's modern synthesis of traditional Japanese and traditional Western Reiki techniques.

In 1997, Rev. Inamoto began teaching Komyo Reiki, his synthesis of these traditional forms, with an emphasis on the spirituality of Reiki practice—a spiritual pathway to Satori (enlightenment). Because of his Buddhist perspective, he encourages meditation as an important element of daily Reiki practice and offers not only traditional methods (including Hatsurei-ho) to activate Reiki energy within, but also Anapanasati, a Buddhist meditation that may be easily learned to support the attainment of "mindfulness / awareness of being in the present moment, Now and Here."[6] His classes for Western Reiki masters also include instruction in hand placement, self- and client treatment, the Reiki symbols, distant healing, and Komyo Reiki reiju.

Rev. Inamoto is comfortable speaking and writing English, and so includes translations of the Gokai (Reiki principles), the Hikkei, the Meiji Tenno Gyosei (Meiji Emporer's poems adopted by Mikao Usui for contemplation), and the Usui Memorial in his instructional manual as resources for his students. He has adopted the following motto as a spiritual practice for Komyo Reiki Kai, *"Homerare temo / Kenasare temo / Heizen to ayume / ayume!"* which is translated as "Go placidly in the midst of praise or blame!" The motto connotes "nonattachment and transcendence of the world of duality."[7]

He encourages those who wish to increase their Reiki energy level to cultivate and develop their spirituality; "to receive reiju (attunement) as often as possible"; and to do daily meditation, with hands in gassho, twice daily.[8]

To contact Rev. Inamoto, you may write an e-mail to him in English at komyo100@yahoo.co.jp. For information regarding his upcoming classes in North America, please contact Komyo Reiki teacher Elyssa Matthews at kokoro@dsl.ca.

THE RADIANCE TECHNIQUE AND RADIANT PEACE ASSOCIATES INTERNATIONAL

Dr. Barbara Ray claims to have been taught seven levels of Reiki by Hawayo Takata in the year before her death. The organization she founded presents these in a seven-level class sequence as Authentic Reiki (also Real Reiki) to distinguish this system from that taught by Takata to the other twenty-one traditional Usui Reiki masters. Since 1982, Ray has published more than half a dozen books describing the Radiance Technique energy system, which emphasizes stress management and personal growth and development; her first book, *The 'Reiki' Factor in The Radiance Technique* is regarded as the best introduction to this system. Practitioners of traditional Usui Reiki who are interested in learning this system are required to start at level one.

For more information, visit the association's website, www.trtia.org, or e-mail them at trtia@trtia.org.

TRADITIONAL JAPANESE REIKI (TJR) OR "USUI-DO"

In 1971, on a trip to Morocco, Dave King met an elderly Japanese man named Onuki Yuji, who had learned healing techniques he attributed to Mikao Usui and to Eguchi Toshihiro. Impressed with King's knowledge of qigong, Yuji taught him some of these techniques, and King continued to practice them. Two decades later, King was invited to a "First Degree Reiki" class in Canada, where he then lived. He was surprised to hear Usui portrayed as a Christian monk, and this set him wondering what really happened. He traveled to Tokyo to see if he could locate the Usui Memorial that Yuji had described to him. He was rewarded for his efforts by an encounter with a man whose father had studied with Usui in 1923. This gentleman showed him a scroll on which the original Reiki principles, the Gainen, had been brushed in Usui's own hand.

On subsequent visits to Japan, King attended a workshop led by Japanese Reiki Master Toshitaka Mochizuki (the founder of the Vortex school, described below); visited with an elderly gentleman named Tatsumi, who had studied with Dr. Hayashi in the late 1920s and early 1930s; and was introduced to two Tendai Buddhist nuns who had followed Usui during the last six years of his life.

Through these sources, King and his research partner, Melissa Riggal, came to a different understanding of Reiki history, which emphasized Mikao Usui's Buddhist spiritual practice and recorded his first use of the Reiki method in or around 1914 and the establishment of his school, Usui Reiki Ryoho, in Tokyo in 1921. This inspired them to create a system of Reiki that they believed was

235

more historically accurate and faithful to Usui's original focus. They first began teaching this system as Traditional Japanese Reiki in 1995.[9]

Traditional Japanese Reiki masters emphasize practice of Usui-do, a way of life guided by the Gainen, or Reiki principles. They teach different hand positions for Reiki level I, which follow the energy meridians as described by Chinese medicine. They teach the same distant-healing symbols for Reiki level II, using tracings of the Reiki symbols drawn in Usui's hand and providing one attunement with each symbol. They teach level III as self-empowerment, and invite level III practitioners to commit to teaching, but do not require it; the commitment asked to become a teacher is not one of money, but of time to apprentice and learn well.

Two books provide valuable perspective on Traditional Japanese Reiki. Dave King's *O-Sensei: A View of Mikao Usui* (ID#356445, www.lulupress.com, 2006) shares the view of Mariko Obaasan, one of the Buddhist nuns who closely followed Mikao Usui and joined with him in his original practice of recitation of the Gainen (the Reiki principles), even before the element of "hand healing" was added. Another book, *Reiki, the True Story: An Exploration of Usui Reiki* by Don Beckett, a longtime correspondent of Dave King's, reiterates some of this early history and expands upon key elements with new details.

Dave King now lives in China, where he continues to do research. He also occasionally travels to Canada to teach Traditional Japanese Reiki to interested students. For more information, visit his website, www.usui-do.org, or send an e-mail to him at usuido@usui-do.org.

USUI REIKI RYOHO

When Japanese Reiki Master Hiroshi Doi first visited the West in August, 1999, he brought with him a great gift: knowledge of the history, techniques, and attunement methods that had been passed down from one generation to the next within the Usui Reiki Ryoho Gakkai, the learning society that was formed during the early 1920s for the purpose of offering instruction and practice in Usui Reiki. Doi, who is a member of the Gakkai, requested and received permission to share this historical information freely from the then chairperson, Mrs. Kimiko Koyama, and he has done so with a generosity of spirit and a gentle wisdom that is gratefully remembered by all who have met him.

Doi described the Gakkai itself as an organization of people who are devoted to the practice of Usui Reiki. They meet monthly, and at each meeting a Shihan (or master) will lead a meditation, offer a reiju (or empowerment), and provide some instruction and supervision of practice. Those who are interested in joining must be invited to a meeting by a current member; if the individual continues to be intent on learning Reiki, a lifetime commitment (expressed by payment of a small fee) is required. Despite Mikao Usui's intention to share Reiki with the public at large, soon after World War II it became necessary for the Gakkai to operate as a secret society, and it continues to do so today.[10]

Progression from practitioner to master within the Gakkai requires great dedication and often takes many years. Students begin as Shoden and must fulfill stringent requirements to advance to Okuden level; very few progress to Shinpiden level. As a result, many Japanese now choose to learn Western style Reiki rather than pursue membership within the Gakkai. Sadly, this has meant that the membership has decreased in numbers.

Although the Gakkai itself is closed to us, Doi continues to travel the world, teaching the history of Usui Reiki and many of the historical techniques as part of Gendai Reiki, his modern synthesis of traditional Japanese and Western techniques (see Gendai Reiki, page 231). In Australia, two of his students, Frans and Bronwen Stiene, have decided to teach Usui Reiki Ryoho techniques exclusively, even though Doi has made clear that these techniques are historic, rather than current. Even so, many people feel quite happy to learn the Usui Reiki Ryoho techniques as their entry onto the Reiki path, and the Stienes are popular teachers in Australia, where they live. Recently, they have begun traveling to teach Usui Reiki Ryoho workshops in Europe and in the United States. To learn more, visit their website, www.reiki.net.au, or e-mail them at info@ reiki.net.au.

VORTEX REIKI

This form of traditional Reiki was created by Toshitaka Mochizuki, the author of *Iyashi No Te* ("Healing of Hands" or "Healing Hands"), the first book about

Reiki published in Japanese (1995). Mochizuki credits another author, Takichi Tsukida, as his source for historical information about the life and teachings of Mikao Usui. Tsukida acknowledges one particular follower of the Usui Reiki method, Toshihiro Eguchi, who was himself a famous healer, as someone who influenced and helped to shape early Reiki practice, so that it included palm healing.

Mochizuki is not a member of the Usui Reiki Gakkai, although he maintains close contact with the group. He teaches Vortex Reiki on a monthly basis in Tokyo, Japan, with the help of other Reiki masters, so that each student may still receive personal attention and be guided in their initial practice. He offers instruction in the first and second degrees of Reiki in a weekend class. For more information, visit www.reiki-japan.net or send an e-mail to reiki@reiki.ne.jp.

The creators of the various forms of Reiki described above all attempt to live by the values recommended by Mikao Usui: peace, serenity, gratitude, integrity, and kindness. They also acknowledge their own humanity and the spiritual evolution they have experienced as they have practiced Reiki. This humility and generosity of spirit enables them to serve well as both teachers and practitioners. Because the forms of traditional Reiki they present have been found to provide effective healing, they are sought out as instructors around the world.

If you are interested in further exploration of any of these forms of traditional Reiki, please have a treatment by a practitioner before deciding to sign up for a class. The experience of the energy that flows through the practitioner's hands will tell you more about whether or not this form of Reiki is for you than anything you can read in a book. If possible, talk to the person who will be your teacher. Finally, reflect on what you have experienced and what you have been told. Listen to your heart. Let the last word be spoken by the God within you.

Appendix 3

RESOURCES

REIKI ORGANIZATIONS AND ASSOCIATIONS

In one class I described the Reiki path as one for rugged spiritual individu-alists. The students laughed, recognizing how important an absolute fidelity to their own inner guidance had been in bringing them to the point where they were learning Reiki. I meant the comment seriously, however. Many tra-ditional Usui-method Reiki practitioners and teachers (including some of the Reiki masters trained by Takata herself) have no affiliation with any formal organization, and yet they practice and teach with a great love and enthusi-asm for Reiki.

Organizations do exist for those who feel a desire for professional fellow-ship or a focus on service. If you would like to become part of a community of Reiki practitioners, contact the following organizations to learn more about the particular purposes they serve. By making an effort to get to know more about these organizations and associations, the practitioner can find others with shared priorities.

International Association of Reiki Professionals, LLC (IARP)
20 Trafalgar Square, Suite 405
Nashua, NH 03063
(866) 888-0856
www.iarpreiki.org
Focus: Professional standards and support services; liability insurance; membership directory; publications

The International Center for Reiki Training
21421 Hilltop Street, Unit #28
Southfield, MI 48033
(800) 332-8112; (248) 948-8112
www.reiki.org
center@reiki.org
Focus: Community education; teaching of Usui-Tibetan Reiki and Karuna Reiki; global healing; world peace

Reiki Outreach International
P.O. Box 191156
San Diego, CA 92119-1156
www.annieo.com/reikioutreach/index.htm
ann@annieo.com
Focus: Humanitarian service; world healing

The Reiki Alliance
204 N. Chestnut Street
Kellogg, ID 83837
208-783-3535
www.reikialliance.com
internationaloffice@reikialliance.com
Focus: Preservation of Usui Shiki Ryoho methods of healing and instruction, as taught by Hawayo Takata to her students; recognition of Phyllis Furumoto, granddaughter of Hawayo Takata as "lineage bearer" and spiritual leader; fellowship. See also www.usuishikiryohoreiki.com.

The Radiance Technique International Association, Inc.
P.O. Box 40570
St. Petersburg, FL 33743
www.trtia.org
trtia@trtia.org
Focus: Teaching of the Radiance Technique; peace projects

SUPPORTING ASSOCIATIONS

Health-care practitioners who learn Reiki and want to integrate it into their professional practice may find the following associations useful for networking, referrals, and other forms of support.

American Association of Naturopathic Physicians
4435 Wisconsin Avenue NW, Suite 403
Washington, DC 20016
(866) 538-2267
www.naturopathic.org
member.services@naturopathic.org

American Holistic Medicine Association
23366 Commerce Park, Suite 101B
Beachwood, OH 44122
(216) 292-6644
www.holisticmedicine.org
info@holisticmedicine.org

American Holistic Nurses Association
323 N. San Francisco Street, Suite 201
Flagstaff, AZ 86001
(800) 278-2462
www.ahna.org
info@ahna.org

American Holistic Veterinary Association
2214 Old Emmorton Road
Bel Air, MD 21025
(410) 569-0795
www.ahvma.org
office@ahvma.org

The American Massage Therapy Association
500 Davis Street, Suite 900
Evanston, IL 60201-4695
(877) 905-2700
www.amtamassage.org
info@amtamassage.org

Associated Bodywork and Massage Professionals
25188 Genesee Trail Road
Golden, CO 80401
(800) 458-2267
(303) 674-8478
www.abmp.com
expectmore@abmp.com

National Association of Massage Therapists
P.O. Box 293
Casanova, VA 20139
(800) 776-6268
www.namtonline.com
info@namtonline.com

STATE LICENSING ORGANIZATIONS

Reiki practitioners interested in establishing a professional practice who do not have existing qualifying credentials in another health-care field may want to explore the option of becoming a massage therapist with Reiki as a featured modality. As of this writing, most states have specific licensing requirements for massage therapy; other states have legislation pending.

In order to find out the most current licensing requirements in your state or a state to which you are considering moving, please visit the website of Associated Bodywork & Massage Professionals (www.abmp.com) and click on "Careers." This link brings up a map of the United States, which links to a table providing individual state regulatory and regulatory board contact information. The ABMP constantly updates this information, both online and in their membership magazine, *Massage & Bodywork*.

ON ORDINATION TO MINISTRY

As an alternative to becoming licensed as a massage therapist, the Reiki practitioner who wishes to establish a professional practice may consider becoming ordained as a minister, either in the religion of his choice or in a nondenominational church. The Universal Life Church, which attracted former President

Lyndon Baines Johnson to its membership, is one such nondenominational church. The Universal Life Church, headquartered at 601 3rd Street, Modesto, CA 95351, encourages anyone interested in exploring this opportunity online to visit www.ulc.net, or to send a letter of inquiry to ULC Online, P.O. Box 1034, Folsom, CA 95763-1034. The organization can also be contacted by phone: (209) 527-8111; or (916) 265-2468.

Becoming ordained as a minister allows the practitioner to legally provide the comfort of healing touch, as clergy are allowed this privilege in ministering to the sick and the dying under the Constitution, which separates church and state.

SOURCES FOR TREATMENT TABLES AND OTHER SUPPLIES

Best Massage.com—TAO Trading Corp.
1419 W. Howard Street
Chicago, IL 60626
(773) 764-6542
www.bestmassage.com

Blue Ridge Tables
915-A Highway 45
Corinth, MS 38834
(800) 447-2723
www.blueridgetables.com
blueridge@dixie-net.com

Custom Craftworks
760 Bailey Hill Road
P.O. Box 24621
Eugene, OR 97402-5451
(800) 627-2387
www.customcraftworks.com
info@customcrafts.com

Robert Hunter Bodywork Tables
Robert Hunter & Company
910 SE Stark Street

Portland, OR 97214
(800) 284-3988
www.roberthunter.com
sales@roberthunter.com

Massage Central
12235 Santa Monica Boulevard
West Los Angeles, CA 90025
(888) 818-2040
(310) 826-2209
www.mcla.com
info@mcla.com

Oakworks, Inc.
923 E. Wellspring Road
New Freedom, PA 17349
(800) 558-8850
www.oakworks.com

Stronglite Massage Tables
369 S. Orange Street, #7
Salt Lake City, UT 84104
(800) 289-5487
www.stronglite.com
info@stronglite.com

PROFESSIONAL CODES OF ETHICS

The Associated Bodywork & Massage Professionals (ABMP) and International Association of Reiki Professionals (IARP) codes of ethics are good models for professional conduct in the treatment-room setting.

ABMP CODE OF ETHICS

As a member of Associated Bodywork & Massage Professionals, I hereby pledge to abide by the ABMP Code of Ethics as outlined below.

Client Relationships

- I shall endeavor to serve the best interests of my clients at all times and to provide the highest quality service possible.

- I shall maintain clear and honest communications with my clients and shall keep client communications confidential.

- I shall acknowledge the limitations of my skills and, when necessary, refer clients to the appropriate qualified health care professional.

- I shall in no way instigate or tolerate any kind of sexual advance while acting in the capacity of a massage, bodywork, somatic therapy or esthetic practitioner.

Professionalism

- I shall maintain the highest standards of professional conduct, providing services in an ethical and professional manner in relation to my clientele, business associates, health care professionals, and the general public.

- I shall respect the rights of all ethical practitioners and will cooperate with all health care professionals in a friendly and professional manner.

- I shall refrain from the use of any mind-altering drugs, alcohol, or intoxicants prior to or during professional sessions.

- I shall always dress in a professional manner, proper dress being defined as attire suitable and consistent with accepted business and professional practice.

- I shall not be affiliated with or employed by any business that utilizes any form of sexual suggestiveness or explicit sexuality in its advertising or promotion of services, or in the actual practice of its services.

Scope of Practice/Appropriate Techniques

- I shall provide services within the scope of the ABMP definition of massage, bodywork, somatic therapies and skin care, and the limits of my training. I will not employ those massage, bodywork or skin care techniques for which I have not had adequate training and shall represent my education, training, qualifications and abilities honestly.

- I shall be conscious of the intent of the services that I am providing and shall be aware of and practice good judgment regarding the application of massage, bodywork or somatic techniques utilized.

- I shall not perform manipulations or adjustments of the human skeletal structure, diagnose, prescribe or provide any other service, procedure or therapy which requires a license to practice chiropractic, osteopathy, physical therapy, podiatry, orthopedics, psychotherapy, acupuncture, dermatology, cosmetology, or any other profession or branch of medicine unless specifically licensed to do so.

- I shall be thoroughly educated and understand the physiological effects of the specific massage, bodywork, somatic or skin care techniques utilized in order to determine whether such application is contraindicated and/or to determine the most beneficial techniques to apply to a given individual. I shall not apply massage, bodywork, somatic or skin care techniques in those cases where they may be contraindicated without a written referral from the client's primary care provider.

Image/Advertising Claims

- I shall strive to project a professional image for myself, my business or place of employment, and the profession in general.

- I shall actively participate in educating the public regarding the actual benefits of massage, bodywork, somatic therapies and skin care.

- I shall practice honesty in advertising, promote my services ethically and in good taste, and practice and/or advertise only those techniques for which I have received adequate training and/or certification. I shall not make false claims regarding the potential benefits of the techniques rendered.

© Associated Bodywork & Massage Professionals

IARP CODE OF ETHICS

The Registered Reiki Practitioner (RP)/Registered Reiki Master Practitioner and Teacher (RMT) agrees to:

1. Abide by a vow of confidentiality. Any information that is discussed within the context of a Reiki session is confidential between the client and practitioner.
2. Provide a safe and comfortable area for sessions or classes and work to provide an empowering and supportive environment for clients and students.
3. Always treat clients and students with the utmost respect and honor.
4. Have a pure and clear intention to offer your services for the highest healing good of the client and highest potential of the student.

247

5. Provide a brief oral or written description of what happens during a session and what to expect before a client's initial session. Provide a clear written description of subjects to be taught during each level of Reiki prior to class and list what the student will be able to do after taking the class.

6. Be respectful of all others' Reiki views and paths.

7. Educate clients/students on the value of Reiki and explain that sessions do not guarantee a cure, nor are they a substitute for qualified medical or professional care. Reiki is one part of an integrative healing or wellness program.

8. Suggest a consultation or referral for clients to qualified licensed professionals (medical doctor, licensed therapist, etc.) when appropriate.

9. Never diagnose or prescribe. Never suggest that the client/student change prescribed treatment or interfere with the treatment of a licensed health care provider.

10. Be sensitive to the boundary needs of individual clients and students.

11. Never ask clients to disrobe (unless in the context of a licensed massage therapy session at the client's option). Do not touch the genital area or breasts. Practice hands-off healing of these areas if treatment is needed.

12. Be working to create harmony and friendly cooperation between Reiki Practitioners/ Master Teachers in the community and represent the IARP in a most professional manner.

13. Act as a beacon in your community by doing the best job possible.

14. Work to empower your students to heal themselves and to encourage and assist them in the development of their work with Reiki or their Reiki practices.

15. Be actively working on your own healing so as to embody and fully express the essence of Reiki in everything that you do.

IARP Registered Reiki Practitioners and Teachers strive to provide the highest quality Reiki experience and abide by the IARP Code of Ethics.

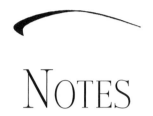

NOTES

PREFACE TO THE REVISED EDITION

1. Tadao Yamaguchi, *Light on the Origins of Reiki: A Handbook for Practicing the Original Reiki of Usui and Hayashi* (Twin Lakes, Wis.: Lotus Press, 2007), 61.

2. Ibid., 68.

3. Ibid., 17.

4. Marianne Streich, "How Hawayo Takata Practiced and Taught Reiki," *Reiki News Magazine* 6, no. 1 (Spring 2007): 11.

5. Helen J. Haberly, *Reiki: Hawayo Takata's Story* (Olney, Md.: Archedigm Publications, 1990), 31.

6. Fran Brown, *Living Reiki: Takata's Teachings* (Mendocino, Calif.: LifeRhythm, 1992), 333–39.

7. John Harvey Gray and Lourdes Gray. *Hand to Hand: The Longest-Practicing Reiki Master Tells His Story* (Philadelphia: Xlibris Corporation, 2002), www.xlibris.com, 30.

8. Frank Arjava Petter, Tadao Yamaguchi, and Chujiro Hayashi, *The Hayashi Reiki Manual: Traditional Japanese Healing Techniques from the Founder of the Western Reiki System* (Twin Lakes, Wis.: Lotus Press, 2004), 27.

9. Haberly, *Reiki: Hawayo Takata's Story,* 42.

10. Ibid., 43.

CHAPTER 1. A HEALING METHOD "FOR THE GOOD OF HUMANKIND"

1. Mikao Usui, *Reiki Ryoho Hikkei*, trans. Christine M. Grimm, in Frank Arjava Petter, *The Original Reiki Handbook of Dr. Mikao Usui* (Twin Lakes, Wis.: Lotus Press, 1999). See also "Excerpt from the *Reiki Ryoho Hikkei*," *Reiki*

News Magazine 5, no. 2 (Summer 2006): 18–23, which features portions of the Hikkei translation originally included by Rev. Hyakuten Inamoto in his Komyo Reiki instructional manual.

2. Hyakuten Inamoto, "Excerpt from the *Reiki Ryoho Hikkei*," 20.

3. Frank Arjava Petter, *Reiki Fire: New Information about the Origins of the Reiki Power: A Complete Manual* (Twin Lakes, Wis.: Lotus Press, 1997), 29.

4. Hyakuten Inamoto, "Excerpt from the *Reiki Ryoho Hikkei*," 20.

5. Ibid.

6. Ibid.

CHAPTER 2. REIKI IN THE CONTEXT OF OUR TIME

1. Mikao Usui, *Reiki Ryoho Hikkei,* trans. Christine M. Grimm, in Frank Arjava Petter, *The Original Reiki Handbook of Dr. Mikao Usui* (Twin Lakes, Wis.: Lotus Press, 1999). See also "Excerpts from the *Reiki Ryoho Hikkei*," *Reiki News Magazine* 5, no. 2 (Summer 2006): 18–23, which features portions of the Hikkei translation made by Rev. Hyakuten Inamoto for his Komyo Reiki instructional manual. In addition, excerpts of the Hikkei have been published in instructional manuals and conference handouts prepared for Mr. Hiroshi Doi, who teaches workshops on the historical Usui Reiki Ryoho techniques.

2. Mr. Hiroshi Doi, in his translation of the Usui Memorial, specifies that Mikao Usui began his meditation and fast on Mount Kurama in March 1922. This translation is included in Rick R. Rivard and Tom Rigler's *Usui Reiki Ryoho: Shoden, Okuden, and Shinpiden Japanese Reiki Workshop Manual* (Toronto and Baltimore: Reiki-ho Resources, 1999), Shoden-6.

3. Frank Arjava Petter, *Reiki: The Legacy of Dr. Usui* (Twin Lakes, Wis.: Lotus Press, 1999), 26.

4. Mr. Hiroshi Doi, at various international conferences, has mentioned his discovery of an early twentieth-century book called *A Path to Soundness,* by Dr. Suzuki Bizan. Hyakuten Inamoto provides more details in his manual, *Komyo Reiki Kai: Reiki Healing Art* (Kyoto, Japan: Komyo Reiki Kai, 2002), 24.

5. Frank Arjava Petter, Tadao Yamaguchi, and Chujiro Hayashi, *The Hayashi Reiki Manual: Traditional Japanese Healing Techniques from the Founder of the Western Reiki System* (Twin Lakes, Wis.: Lotus Press, 2004).

6. William L. Rand, *Reiki: The Healing Touch; First and Second Degree Manual.* (Southfield, Mich.: Vision Publication, 2005).

7. John Harvey Gray and Lourdes Gray, *Hand to Hand: The Longest-Practicing Reiki Master Tells His Story,* with Steven McFadden and Elisabeth Clark (Philadelphia: Xlibris Corporation, 2002), www.xlibris.com.

8. Helen J. Haberly, *Reiki: Hawayo Takata's Story* (Olney, Md.: Archedigm Publications, 1990), 26.

9. Petter, Yamaguchi, and Hayashi, *The Hayashi Reiki Manual,* 34, 63.

10. Ibid., 36.

11. Marianne Streich, "How Takata Practiced and Taught Reiki," *Reiki News Magazine* 6, no. 1 (Spring 2007), 11.

12. Alice Furumoto, *Reiki: The Usui System of Natural Healing,* ed. Paul David Mitchell, 2nd rev. ed. (Coeur d'Alere, Ind.: The Reiki Alliance, 1985). 1st ed. 1982; Phyllis Furumoto, 1st revised edition, 1985. Citation is to The Reiki Alliance edition.

13. Rev. Beth Gray provided a copy of this article to her Reiki I students during the late 1980s.

14. William Lee Rand, "Takata's Handouts," *Reiki News Magazine* 8, no. 2 (Summer 2009): 58–63. Article cites handouts contributed by Alice Picking.

15. Hawayo Takata, *Takata Speaks, Vol. 1: Reiki Stories,* audiotape of Reiki master training classes of Hawayo Takata conducted in 1976. (Rindge, NH: The John Harvey Gray Center for Reiki Healing, n.d.)

16. Furumoto, *Reiki: The Usui System of Natural Healing,* 3.

17. Gray and Gray, *Hand to Hand,* 93.

18. Haberly, *Reiki: Hawayo Takata's Story,* 52, 56, 57.

19. Rand, "Takata's Handouts."

20. Larry Arnold and Sandy Nevius, *The Reiki Handbook: A Manual for Students and Therapists of the Usui Shiki Ryoho System of Healing* (Harrisburg, Pa.: PSI Press, 1982).

21. Diane Stein, *Essential Reiki: A Complete Guide to an Ancient Healing Art* (Berkeley: Crossing Press, 1995).

22. Frank Arjava Petter, *Reiki Fire: New Information about the Origins of the Reiki Power: A Complete Manual* (Twin Lakes, Wis.: Lotus Press, 1997), 18, 21.

CHAPTER 3. BASICS OF PRACTICE

1. Helen J. Haberly, *Reiki: Hawayo Takata's Story* (Olney, Md.: Archedigm Publications, 1990), 26.

CHAPTER 6. THE ORIGIN OF REIKI HEALING

1. Frank Arjava Petter, Tadao Yamaguchi, and Chujiro Hayashi, *The Hayashi Reiki Manual: Traditional Japanese Healing Techniques from the Founder of the Western Reiki System* (Twin Lakes, Wis.: Lotus Press, 2004), 13.

2. Helen J. Haberly, *Reiki: Hawayo Takata's Story* (Olney, Md.: Archedigm Publications, 1990), 18.

3. Fran Brown, *Living Reiki: Takata's Teachings* (Mendocino, Calif.: LifeRhythm, 1992), 24.

4. Haberly, *Reiki: Hawayo Takata's Story,* 23–26.

5. Ibid., 25–26.

6. Ibid., 27–29.

7. Ibid., 31.

8. Brown, *Living Reiki: Takata's Teachings,* 38.

9. Ibid., 38–39.

10. Although neither Helen Haberly, Hawayo Takata's official biographer, nor Fran Brown, one of her master students, provides this detail in their books about Takata's life and practice, I remember my teacher, Takata-trained Reiki Master Rev. Beth Gray, describing this in my Reiki I class in March 1987 and at each of the Reiki I classes at which I assisted during the next five years.

11. Marianne Streich provides more details on Takata's instruction of her master students in "How Hawayo Takata Practiced and Taught Reiki," *Reiki News Magazine* 6, no. 1 (Spring 2007): 18.

12. Larry Arnold and Sandy Nevius, *The Reiki Handbook: A Manual for Students and Therapists of the Usui Shiki Ryoho System of Healing* (Harrisburg, Pa.: PSI Press, 1982).

13. Diane Stein, *Essential Reiki: A Complete Guide to an Ancient Healing Art* (Freedom, Calif.: Crossing Press, 1995).

14. Haberly, *Reiki: Hawayo Takata's Story,* 52.

15. Frank Arjava Petter, *Reiki Fire: New Information about the Origins of the Reiki Power; A Complete Manual* (Twin Lakes, Wis.: Lotus Press, 1997), 22.

16. Ibid., 26.

17. Ibid., 28.

18. Hyakuten Inamoto, *Komyo Reiki Kai: Reiki Healing Art* (Kyoto, Japan: Komyo Reiki Kai, 2002), 13-18. Reprint of Rev. Inamoto's translation used by permission.

19. Tadao Yamaguchi, *Light on the Origins of Reiki: A Handbook for Practicing the Original Reiki of Usui and Hayashi* (Twin Lakes, Wis.: Lotus Press, 2007), 17.

20. Hyakuten Inamoto, "Excerpt from the *Reiki Ryoho Hikkei*" *Reiki News Magazine* 5, no. 2 (Summer 2006), 13.

21. Alice Furumoto, *Reiki: The Usui System of Natural Healing,* ed. Paul David Mitchell, 2nd rev. ed. (Coeur d'Alere, Ind.: The Reiki Alliance, 1985). 1st ed. 1982; Phyllis Furumoto, 1st revised edition, 1985. Citation is to The Reiki Alliance edition, 1.

22. Ibid.

CHAPTER 7. A METAPHYSICAL APPROACH TO HEALING, HEALTH, AND WELLNESS

1. Helen J. Haberly, *Reiki: Hawayo Takata's Story* (Olney, Md.: Archedigm Publications, 1990), 56–57.

2. Reiki Master Beth Gray enjoyed making her students laugh with this catchy rhyme that stayed in our minds long after the Reiki I class to remind us that it is usually not in anyone's best interests to repress negative emotions, especially over a long period of time.

3. Both of these books are out of print, but they are well worth searching for as "used books" on eBay or Amazon.

4. Louise L. Hay, *You Can Heal Your Life* (Santa Monica: Hay House, Inc., 1984). Millions of copies of this book have been sold around the world since it was first published, and it is available in movie form as well. Louise L. Hay, *You Can Heal Your Life—The Movie* (www.youcanhealyourlifemovie.com/) 2007.

5. Hay, *You Can Heal Your Life*, 72.

6. Louise L. Hay, *You Can Heal Your Body* (Santa Monica, Calif.: Hay House, 1982), 2.

7. Joseph LeDoux, interview by Michael Grillen, *Good Morning America*, ABC television network, March 11, 1997.

8. e.e. cummings, "Since Feeling Is First" *Modern American Poetry*, ed. Louise Untermeyer (New York: Harcourt, Brace & World, 1962), 476.

9. "Change Your Life in a Heartbeat," sidebar in *Natural Health* (April 1997): 103.

10. Haberly, *Reiki: Hawayo Takata's Story,* 51.

11. Ibid., 52.

CHAPTER 8. PRACTICAL HUMAN ANATOMY

1. Stephen Ceci, interview by Michael Grillen, *Good Morning America,* ABC television network, March 11, 1997.

CHAPTER II. REIKI LEVEL II: AN OVERVIEW OF THE ADVANCED COURSE

1. Larry Arnold and Sandy Nevius, *The Reiki Handbook: A Manual For Students and Therapists of the Usui Shiki Ryoho System of Healing* (Harrisburg, Pa.: PSI Press, 1982), 67.

APPENDIX I. HAWAYO TAKATA'S STORY
OF MIKAO USUI

1. John Morrow, telephone conversation with the author, June 3, 2009.

2. Tadao Yamaguchi, *Light on the Origins of Reiki: A Handbook for Practicing the Original Reiki of Usui and Hayashi* (Twin Lakes, Wis.: Lotus Press, 2007), 61.

3. John Harvey Gray and Lourdes Gray, *Hand to Hand: The Longest-Practicing Reiki Master Tells His Story* (Philadelphia: Xlibris Corporation, 2002), www.xlibris .com.

4. Hyakuten Inamoto, "Excerpt from the *Reiki Ryoho Hikkei*" *Reiki News Magazine* 5, no. 2 (Summer 2006), 13.

APPENDIX 2. EXPLORATIONS: BOUNDLESS REIKI,
BOUNDLESS LEARNING

1. "About The International Center for Reiki Training," www.reiki.org/AboutICRT/ AboutICRT.html.

2. Hiroshi Doi, *Iyashino Gendai Reiki-ho: Modern Reiki Method for Healing*, ed. Rick Rivard and Miyuki Iwasaki, trans. Akiko Kawarai Mari Marchand, Hiroko and Phillip Kelly, Emiko Arai, Yukio Miura, Yuko Okamoto (Coquitlam, BC, Canada: Fraser, 2000), 8.

3. Ibid., 33–37.

4. This information was shared by Rev. Hyakuten Inamoto during a Komyo Reiki workshop held in Toronto, Canada, in October 2006.

5. Tadao Yamaguchi, *Light on the Origins of Reiki: A Handbook for Practicing the Original Reiki of Usui and Hayashi* (Twin Lakes, Wis.: Lotus Press, 2007), 18–19.

6. Hyakuten Inamoto, personal correspondence, November 1, 2009.

7. Hyakuten Inamoto, *Komyo Reiki Kai: Reiki Healing Art* (Kyoto, Japan: Komyo Reiki Kai, 2002), 11.

8. Ibid, 23.

9. Hiroshi Doi, "Usui Reiki Ryoho International Workshop 2002" (lecture and conference proceedings, Toronto, Canada, September 28, 2002).

10. William Lee Rand, "Takata's Handouts," *Reiki News Magazine* 8, no. 2 (Summer 2009): 63.

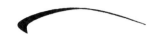

RECOMMENDED READING AND LISTENING

Arnold, Larry, and Sandy Nevius. *The Reiki Handbook: A Manual for Students and Therapists of the Usui Shiki Ryoho System.* Harrisburg: PSI Press, 1982.

Beckett, Don. *Reiki: The True Story; An Exploration of Usui Reiki.* Berkeley: Frog Books, 2009.

Brown, Fran. *Living Reiki: Takata's Teachings.* Mendocino, Calif.: Life Rhythm, 1992.

Doi, Hiroshi. *Iyashino Gendai Reiki-ho: Modern Reiki Method for Healing.* Edited by Rick Rivard and Miyuki Iwasaki. Translated by Akiko Kawarai, Mari Marchand, Hiroko and Phillip Kelly, Emiko Arai, Yukio Miura, and Yuko Okamoto. Coquitlam, BC, Canada: Fraser, 2000.

Gray, John Harvey, and Lourdes Gray. *Hand to Hand: The Longest-Practicing Reiki Master Tells His Story.* With Steven McFadden and Elisabeth Clark. Philadelphia: Xlibris Corporation 2002. www.xlibris.com.

Haberly, Helen. *Reiki: Hawayo Takata's Story.* Olney, Md.: Archedigm, 1990.

Hall, Mari. *Reiki for the Soul: Ten Doorways to Inner Peace.* London: Thorsons Publishers, 2002.

———. *Reiki for the Soul: Doorways to Inner Peace—The Eleventh Door.* Sedona: Infinite Light Healing Studies Center, 2006.

Honervogt, Tanmaya. *Reiki for Emotional Healing.* London: Gaia Books, 2006.

King, Dave. *O-Sensei: A View of Mikao Usui.* Morrisville, N.C.: Dave King/Lulu, 2006. www.book.usui-do.org.

Lübeck, Walter, Frank Arjava Petter, and William Lee Rand. *The Spirit of Reiki: The Complete Handbook of the Reiki System*. Twin Lakes, Wis.: Lotus Press, 2001.

Miles, Pamela. *Reiki: A Comprehensive Guide*. New York: Penguin Group, 2008.

Petter, Frank Arjava. *Reiki Fire: New Information about the Origins of the Reiki Power—A Complete Manual*. Twin Lakes, Wis: Lotus Press, 1997.

———. *Reiki: The Legacy of Dr. Usui*. Twin Lakes, Wis.: Lotus Press, 1998.

Petter, Frank Arjava, and Chetna Kobayashi. *Japanese Reiki Techniques Workshop*. VHS recording. Southfield, Mich: Vision Publications, 2000.

Petter, Frank Arjava, Tadao Yamaguchi, and Chujiro Hayashi. *Hayashi Reiki Manual: Traditional Japanese Healing Techniques from the Founder of the Western Reiki System*. Twin Lakes, Wis.: Lotus Press, 2003.

Rand, William Lee. *Reiki: the Healing Touch; First and Second Degree Manual*. Southfield, Mich.: Vision Publications, 2005.

Ray, Barbara Weber. *The 'Reiki' Factor in the Radiance Technique: Expanded Edition*. St. Petersburg: Radiance Associates, 1992.

Rowland, Amy Z. *Intuitive Reiki for Our Times: Essential Techniques for Enhancing Your Practice*. Rochester, Vt.: Healing Arts Press, 2006.

———. *Reiki for the Heart and Soul: The Reiki Principles as Spiritual Pathwork*. Rochester, Vt.: Healing Arts Press, 2008.

Stein, Diane. *Essential Reiki: A Complete Guide to an Ancient Healing Art*. Berkeley: Crossing Press, 1995.

Stiene, Bronwen, and Frans Stiene. *The Reiki Sourcebook*. Revised edition. Alresford, Hampshire, UK: O Books, 2009.

Takata, Hawayo. *Takata Speaks, Vol. 1: Reiki Stories*. Audiotape of Reiki master training classes of Hawayo Takata conducted in 1976. Rindge, N.H.: The John Harvey Gray Center for Reiki Healing, n.d.

Twan, Anneli. *Early Days of Reiki: Memories of Hawayo Takata*. Hope, BC, Canada: Morning Star Productions, 2005.

Twan, Wanja. *In the Light of a Distant Star: A Spiritual Journey Bringing the Unseen Into the Seen*. Laytonville, Calif.: White Feather Press, 1996.

Usui, Mikao, and Frank Arjava Petter. *The Original Reiki Handbook of Dr. Mikao Usui*. Translated by Christine M. Grimm. Twin Lakes, Wis.: Lotus Press, 1999.

Yamaguchi, Tadao. *Light on the Origins of Reiki: A Handbook for Practicing the Original Reiki of Usui and Hayashi*. Twin Lakes, Wis.: Lotus Press, 2007.

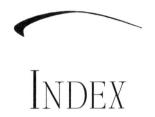

Index

Page numbers in *italics* refer to illustrations.